Monuments of Progress

Latin American and Caribbean Series

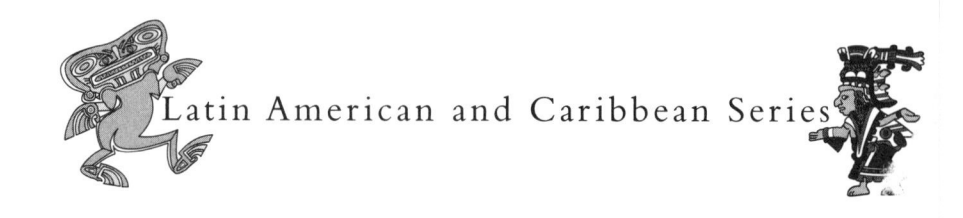

Waking the Dictator
Veracruz, the Struggle for Federalism, and the Mexican Revolution, 1870–1927
Karl B. Koth

The Spirit of Hidalgo
The Mexican Revolution in Coahuila
Suzanne B. Pasztor
Co-published with Michigan State University Press

Clerical Ideology in a Revolutionary Age
The Guadalajara Church and the Idea of the Mexican Nation, 1788–1853
Brian F. Connaughton, translated by Mark Alan Healey
Co-published with University of Colorado Press

Monuments of Progress
Modernization and Public Health in Mexico City, 1876–1910
Claudia Agostoni
Co-published with University Press of Colorado
and Instituto de Investigaciones Históricas, UNAM

Latin American and Caribbean
Christon L. Archer, general editor

University of Calgary Press is pleased to be the publisher of a series that sheds light on historical and cultural topics in Latin America and the Caribbean. Works that challenge the canon in history, literature, and postcolonial studies in this area of the world make this series the only one of its kind in Canada. This series brings to print cutting-edge studies and research that redefine our understanding of historical and current issues in Latin America and the Caribbean.

MONUMENTS OF PROGRESS

Modernization and Public Health in Mexico City, 1876–1910

by Claudia Agostoni

University of Calgary Press
University Press of Colorado
Instituto de Investigaciones Históricas, UNAM

© 2003 Claudia Agostoni. All rights reserved.

University of Calgary Press	University Press of Colorado	Universidad Nacional Autónoma de México
2500 University Drive NW	5589 Arapahoe Ave.	Instituto de Investigaciones Históricas
Calgary, Alberta	Boulder, CO 80303	Ciudad Universitaria
Canada T2N 1N4	U.S.A.	04510 México D.F
www.uofcpress.com	www.upcolorado.com	www.unam.mx/iih

National Library of Canada Cataloguing in Publication Data

Agostoni, Claudia.
  Monuments of progress : modernization and public health in Mexico City, 1876-1910 / by Claudia Agostoni.

  (Latin American and Caribbean series, ISSN 1498-2366 ; 4)
  Includes bibliographical references and index.

  ISBN 1-55238-094-7 (bound) University of Calgary Press
  ISBN 1-55238-103-X (pbk.) University of Calgary Press
  ISBN 0-87081-733-7 (bound) University Press of Colorado
  ISBN 0-87081-734-5 (pbk.) University Press of Colorado

  1. Sanitary engineering—Mexico—Mexico City—History.
  2. Public health—Mexico—Mexico City—History.
  3. Monuments—Mexico—Mexico City—History.
  4. Mexico City (Mexico—History. I. Title. II. Series.

  TD29.M49A36 2003   363.72'0972'53   C2003-910002-2

We acknowledge the financial support of the Government of Canada through the Book Publishing Industry Development Program (BPIDP) for our publishing activities.

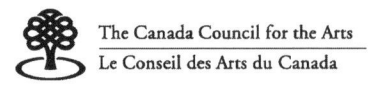

The Canada Council for the Arts
Le Conseil des Arts du Canada

No part of this publication may be reproduced, stored in a retrieval system or transmitted, in any form or by any means, without the prior written consent of the publisher or a licence from The Canadian Copyright Licensing Agency (Access Copyright). For an Access Copyright licence, visit www.accesscopyright.ca or call toll free to 1-800-893-5777.

Printed and bound in Canada by Friesens.
∞ This book is printed on acid-free paper.

Page, cover design, and typesetting by Kristina Schuring.

To Andrea and Ricardo

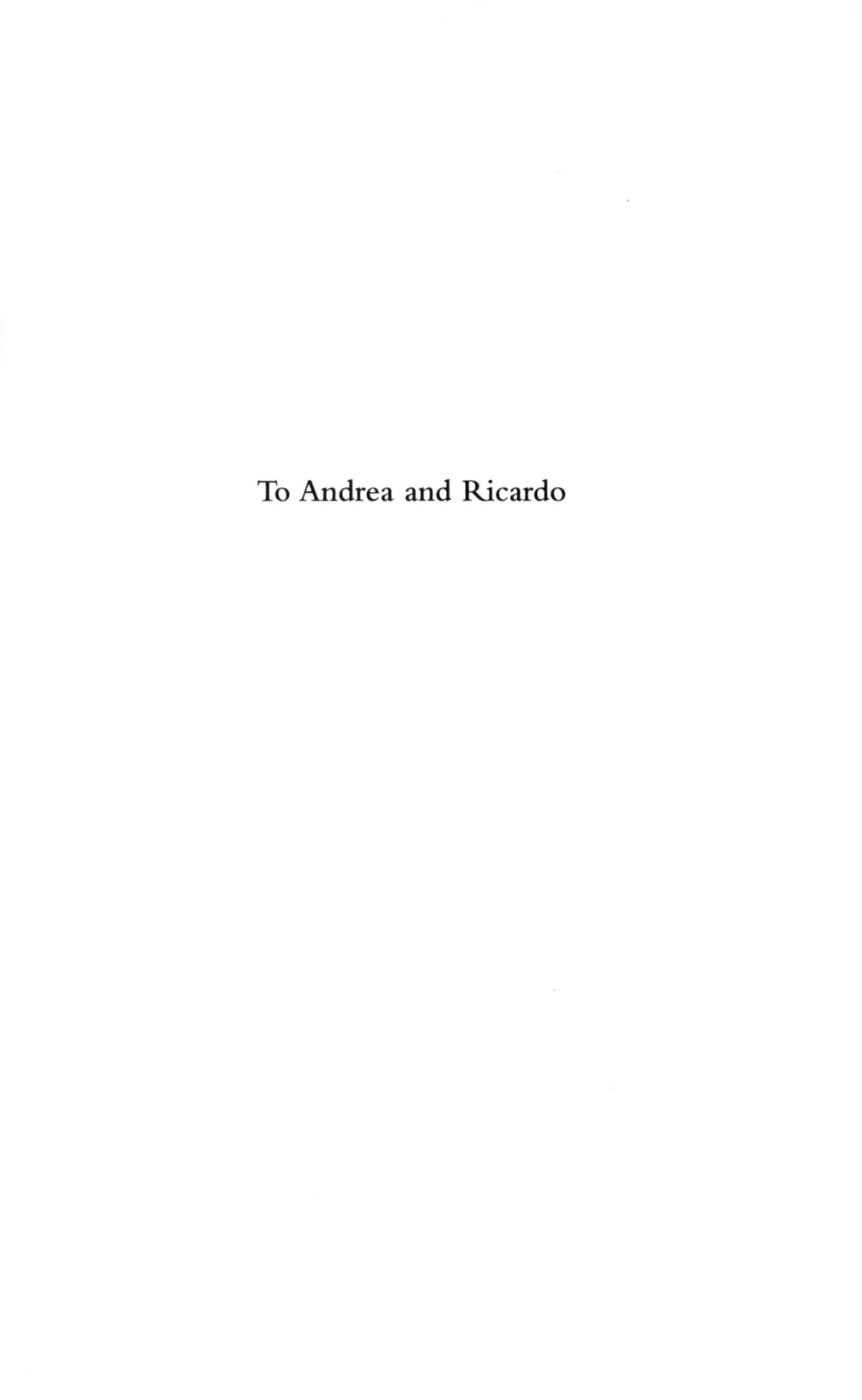

Contents

List of Illustrations	ix
List of Tables	ix
Acknowledgments	x
Introduction	xii

1 Urban Ideas and Projects for Mexico City: The Late Eighteenth Century — 1
  Urban Space and Public Health — 1
  The Unsanitary City — 6
  Viceroy Revillagigedo and Urban Sanitation — 14

2 The Control of the Environment — 23
  The Community of Hygienists — 23
  The Contradictory Proofs of Progress and the City — 26
  Dangerous Elements — 31
  Elements of a Healthy City — 38

3 The Expansion and Diagnosis of the City — 45
  The Expansion of the City — 45
  The Superior Sanitation Council and the Sanitary Code — 57
  The Memoirs of the Sanitary Inspectors — 64
  The Diagnoses of the City — 65

4 The Modern City — 77
  Towards the Secular City — 78
  The Image of the Modern City — 81
  Monuments and the 1877 Decree — 90
  Cuauhtémoc — 97
  Ahuítzotl and Itzcóatl — 100
  Benito Juárez and Independence — 104
  Monumental Space and Cleanliness — 110

5	The Conquest of Water	115
	The Problem: Water	117
	The Drainage System	122
	The Sewage System	130
	Hygiene in the Centennial Celebrations and the Porfirian Inheritance	143

Epilogue	155
Notes	159
Bibliography	195
Index	217

Illustrations

1. José María Velasco, View of the Valley of Mexico from the Hill of Santa Isabel, 1877 — 89
2. Monument to Cuauhtémoc, 1901 — 101
3. Indio Verde on the Calzada de la Viga, 1907 — 102
4. Monument to Benito Juárez, 1911 — 107
5. Monument to Independence — 109
6. Map of the Lakes in the Valley of Mexico, of the Gran Canal and of the Tunnel of the Desagüe — 121
7. The Gran Canal of Desagüe, 1900 — 129
8. The Tunnel of Tequixquiac, 1900 — 140

Tables

1. Expansion of Mexico City, 1858–1910 — 46
2. Mexico City's population by *cuartel* according to the 1890 census — 61
3. Number of premature deaths in Mexico City, 1900–09 — 67
4. Public works undertaken by the government contracted with foreign capital, 1877–1910 — 86
5. Public works undertaken directly by the government, 1877–1910 — 87

Acknowledgments

In writing this book I have become indebted to many people. William Rowe encouraged me to write and supervised the King's College London Ph.D. dissertation where the origins of this book are to be found. The enthusiasm of Solange Alberro, William Beezley, Alberto del Castillo, Charles Hale, Humberto Muñoz, Manuel Perló, Antonio Santoyo, Elisa Speckman, Anne Staples and Guy Thomson, was a crucial stimulus for carrying out further research.

At the Instituto de Investigaciones Históricas of the Universidad Nacional Autónoma de México, I have greatly benefited from the support, and keen interest in my work, from Gisela Von Wobeser and Virginia Guedea. My gratitude also goes to the members of the Seminario de Historia Social y Cultural de la Salud en México (siglos XVIII-XX), with whom I had to opportunity to present and discuss some of the ideas that this book examines.

I also wish to thank the directors and staff at the following libraries and archives: the Archivo Fotográfico of the Instituto de Investigaciones Estéticas of the Universidad Nacional Autónoma de México, the Archivo Histórico del Agua (Mexico), the Archivo Histórico de la Ciudad de México, the Archivo Histórico de la Facultad de Medicina (Mexico), the Archivo Histórico de la Secretaría de Salud (Mexico), the Biblioteca Nacional (Mexico), the Biblioteca Nicolás León (Mexico), El Colegio de México, the Institute of Latin American Studies Library (London), the Science Museum Archive (London), the Fototeca Nacional del Instituto Nacional de Antropología e Historia (Mexico), and the Wellcome Library for the History and Understanding of Medicine (London). My research was funded in part by Mexico's Consejo Nacional de Ciencia y Tecnología and by the University of London, and I am deeply grateful to these institutions.

Portions of chapters 2, 4 and 5 were summarized and included in a different form in the following works: "Salud pública y control social en la ciudad de México a fines del siglo diecinueve," *Historia y grafía* 17 (2001): 73–97; "Mexican Hygienists and the Political and Economic Elite during the Porfirio Díaz Regime. The Case of Mexico City (1876–1910)," in *Les Hygiénistes, enjeux, modèles et pratiques*, sous la direction de Patrice Bourdelais (Paris: Éditions Belin, 2001): 193–210; "Sanitation and Public Works in Late Nineteenth Century Mexico City," *Quipu. Revista Latinoamericana de Historia de las Ciencias y la Tecnología* 12, no. 2 (May–August 1999): 187–201.

I also wish to thank the anonymous reviewers of the University of Calgary Press who read the manuscript closely and made many important critiques and suggestions, and Anna Reid and Alex Larrondo for their invaluable help during the final revision of the manuscript. Finally, I thank Ricardo Salles for his love and support, and Lucille and Giorgio for their kindness and encouragement every step of the way.

Introduction

The period in Mexican history known as the Porfiriato, which is the time of the governments of General Porfirio Díaz (1876–80, 1884–1911) and of General Manuel González (1880–84), has been a topic of study for more than a century. Numerous books, articles and theses have dealt with the issues of state formation and finance, foreign investment, industrialization, agriculture, rural conditions, and the causes and events which led to the 1910 Revolution. This book does not explore any of the issues mentioned above. It concentrates, rather, on particular questions of the environment and public health in Mexico City during the Porfiriato, when the city had less than half a million inhabitants and when the excess of water was regarded as perhaps the most threatening factor to public health and to the very existence of the capital.

The objective of this study is to analyze and discuss why the construction of public works (the drainage system and historical monuments) embodied materially and symbolically the confidence of an era of "order" and "progress" in a context of a largely non-modern society, and why it was thought that the construction of public works would transform the city into a health-giving environment.

During the final decades of the nineteenth century, Mexico City was considered as the most unsanitary place in the world, and this image contrasted sharply with the achievements which statistics ably displayed in the sectors of industry, mines, and commerce. According to the Porfirian elite, the city had two major problems which affected the health of its inhabitants and which threatened its existence: one was the lack of an effective drainage system both in the valley of Mexico and beneath the city, which led to recurrent floods and disease; and the other was the poor hygienic practices among the urban population. This study will therefore explore how public health officials, sanitary engineers and the state intervened in the elaboration of urban projects designed to sanitize the city and to make it conform to the idea that the nation was on the path of progress.

However, the origin of many of the policies dictated during the Porfiriato with the aim of transforming the city's image and sanitary conditions can be traced back to the late eighteenth century, when a critical perception of the city permeated both policies and programs. Therefore, the reasons why the image of the ideal and hygienic city of the late nineteenth century owed a great deal to the Bourbon precedent will also be examined.

The late nineteenth century governing elite attempted to modify the visual aspect and sanitary conditions of the city, and the motives guiding the projects that altered some areas of the capital did not stem solely from the desire to embellish it. To consider that as the guiding element of the discourse of the Porfirian city is far too simplistic. As we shall see, the desire to alter the physiognomy and functioning of the city became a crucial factor in the symbolic legitimation of the Porfirian state, a process that took place at a time during which the capital was reasserting its supremacy over the entire valley of Mexico and the rest of the nation. The fact that a large percentage of national resources, foreign loans and investment were directed towards the city's public works, buildings and historical monuments was congruent with the centralization of economic and political power by the executive branch of government located in the capital. The objective was to make evident, visible and palpable a modern, efficient form of power, to foreigners and nationals alike.

Regarding the construction of public works, and in particular the drainage system, this book will attempt to answer the following questions: Why did the construction of the drainage system become an unavoidable requirement for ordering the urban landscape? What effect would the benefits of this public work have on the visual aspect of the city? How did the altering of the urban landscape below lead to its transformation above ground? What would the implications of this public work be on sanitary conditions? In addition, this book will examine why the construction of the drainage system symbolized the technical, scientific and administrative capacity of a generation of Mexicans who for the first time in the history of the city were able to place under control the menacing natural environment.

The control of the environment, it was thought, would lead to a significant decrease in the high incidence of premature death and disease. One of the prevailing notions of disease causation — the environmentalist theory of disease — forms part of the explanation. Disease, it was argued by many physicians and hygienists, lay in miasmas, in poisonous atmospheric exhalations given off by putrefying carcasses, food and faeces, waterlogged soil, rotting vegetable remains, and other filth in the surroundings. Bad environments, therefore, generated bad air (signalled by stenches), which, in turn, triggered disease. This conception of the etiology of disease began to be challenged during the 1860s and 1870s, and was gradually discredited when the germ theory of disease, developed by the French chemist Louis Pasteur and the German physician Robert Koch, acquired the status of a scientific truth. It is of crucial importance for this study to stress that the breakthroughs in the medical sciences did not immediately cause the dismissal of the miasmatic theory, and that the longstanding view that the environment could cause disease lingered. Therefore, to clean up the environment was not only essential for public health, but also fundamental for the image of the city that the Porfirian elite wished to display.

Public health officials, engineers, and the state bureaucracy all believed that the drainage system was one of the key components that would effectively transform the city. A deodorized, ordered and clean environment became a recurrent motif in the discourse of the modern city elaborated at the time. However, it was also argued that certain social habits and practices of the city dwellers had to change, and therefore public health policies became moral and educational issues.

Within the multiple strategies aimed at attaining a clean and deodorized city, public health officials and hygienists made crucial readings or diagnoses of the urban landscape. The capital city was transformed into a huge laboratory wherein men of science could investigate, dissect and analyze the multiple maladies that afflicted the core of the country. The members of the Superior Sanitation Council (SSC) carried out detailed studies of the unsanitary urban space. Incorporating geography, geology, history, hygiene and economics, and backed by statistics, the sanitary inspectors used the survey techniques of engineers to assess the spatial distribution of disease. These diagnoses of the urban environment, together with the advice and recommendations they prescribed, played a key role in the attempt to reshape the city and the health-endangering social practices of its inhabitants.

The study of public health policy in Mexico City during the Porfiriato uncovers the increasing bureaucratic organization and regulation of society, and reveals the linkage between the scientific discourses of the medical profession and the bureaucratic centralization of state power. Health policies became an extension of the executive power, and the vigorous pursuit of modernization was marked by the erection of barriers and exclusions that stigmatized parts of the urban population as dangerous and vice-ridden. Providing a solution to health problems required state intervention in the form of public works and education.

The construction of the drainage system was not the only requirement for the image of the city. The Paseo de la Reforma — built during the French empire (1864–67) — became the axis for the public display of the Porfirian state, and an official version of history was erected upon it through the construction of historical monuments. Therefore, this study will also examine why the outer surface of the city became the material and symbolic representation of the Porfiriato's achievements. To carry out this task I will not only analyze why it was held that monuments were elements that would give the city a truly metropolitan atmosphere, but also why they symbolized the centralization of political and economic decision-making. I shall try to show how each unveiling and inaugural feast became a celebration of the order and progress made possible by the Díaz government. The historical monuments erected during the Porfiriato reasserted the centralization of power in the capital, presented an official version of history, and transformed the urban landscape above ground, creating boundaries and allegorical landmarks within the city that persist to this day.

The study is composed of five chapters. The first chapter is a historical study which aims at assessing some of the proposals for cleaning up the capital and changing its image during eras previous to the Porfiriato. It tries to show that the origins of the projects that attempted to alter the city's physiognomy and overall functioning predated the 1870s, and that an important impulse for transforming the city emerged during the late colonial period, more precisely during the viceroyalty of the Segundo Conde de

Revillagigedo (1789–94). The chapter examines several key texts of late colonial Mexico City, some of the activities carried out by Viceroy Revillagigedo, and underlines why public health came to be considered a crucial element for the benefit and well-being of the entire society. The impact and force of the Enlightenment reforms was such that they continued to guide many of the projects and proposals that emerged during the course of the nineteenth century, when unprecedented attention was given to the health of the populations and to sanitary reform.

The second chapter explores in detail why, during the late nineteenth century, the geographical location of the city was thought to be a menace for public health, why the capital was prone to suffer from periodic floods, and why the control of water became an unavoidable task for the city's authorities. Physicians and the governing elite believed hat there had to be a correspondence between the progress being achieved — which statistics displayed — and the image of the city. Thus, the environmental elements considered as threatening to health and to the image of the modern city will be identified by looking at diverse texts written during the period by politicians, public health officials and engineers.

Chapter 3 briefly outlines the different phases of urban growth between 1856 and 1910. The focus will be on 1880–1910, years during which the capital grew at an unprecedented pace. It will become apparent that the expansion of the city was neither planned nor supervised, and that it led to the creation of major spatial divisions along social lines. The city became increasingly perceived as formed by two exclusive and distinct entities. The sanitary inspectors of the Superior Sanitation Council maintained that the urban expansion had led to the construction of a modern and hygienic city, but that the health of the entire population was threatened due to the presence of large areas defined as foul-smelling, overcrowded and dangerous. I shall analyze how the sanitary inspectors read the city and how they elaborated detailed diagnoses or medical topographies of the capital. This chapter will also show that the measures put forward to solve its unsanitary conditions embraced not only technical, scientific and administrative aspects, but that they included the inculcation of hygienic practices among the urban population.

Chapter 4 examines some of the architectural innovations of the years 1876 to 1910, and discusses why it was argued that a deodorized and hygienic city had to coexist with a monumental one. Thus, why the erection of monuments was fundamental for the image of city, and why each inauguration became a public manifestation of the centralization of political and economic power in the capital, are issues that will also be explored. At this stage, a further important aspect of the monumental endeavour will also be examined, namely, why the pre-Hispanic past was utilized in national and international settings to promote the stability and progress of the nation.

The last chapter will explore why the construction and completion of the drainage system for the city and valley of Mexico was regarded as the most important public work ever undertaken at the time, and why it was argued that the accomplishment of this secular enterprise had been possible thanks to both the technological advances of the time and the personal commitment of Porfirio Díaz. The chapter also explores why it was hoped that the city was to become, at last, a clean, odour-free urban space, and would no longer suffer from the periodic floods that invaded it, causing the overflow of its sewers, polluting the atmosphere and causing illness and death. Thus, via the construction of a monumental public work, the city would possess, after a long struggle, a healthy and modern environment that previous generations had failed to promote.

1

Urban Ideas and Projects for Mexico City

The Late Eighteenth Century

Urban Space and Public Health

On 8 March 1868, Mexico City's Municipal Council approved a proposal to build a statue to honour the work carried out on behalf of the city by "the best ruler New Spain ever had."[1] The Segundo Conde de Revillagigedo, Don Juan Vicente Güemez, Viceroy of New Spain from 17 October 1789 until 11 July 1794, became identified in the course of the nineteenth century as the man who had accomplished during his brief administration what no other government had achieved: the transformation of the appearance, functioning and sanitary conditions of the city. The arguments for erecting his statue in the avenue named after him stated that it was the duty of the people and of the individual to honour the memory of a benefactor, and Mexico had to fulfill that duty:

> The time has come for the Capital to honor the immense debt of gratitude it has to the ruler that provided Mexico with so many benefits during his brief administration ... Mexico, the capital of one of the most democratic nations of the American continent, remembers that it owes its splendor to that Viceroy and wishes to pay that debt of gratitude and justice.[2]

The immense debt of gratitude that the *capitalinos* owed to Revillagigedo was twofold: first, on account of his efforts to transform the city between 1789 and 1794, and second, on account of the impact of his urban projects upon subsequent governments of Mexico City. Some of the proposals aimed at transforming the urban environment during the late eighteenth century put forward by Viceroy Revillagigedo, by the Regent of the Audiencia, Baltasar Ladrón de Guevara, and by the lawyer Hipólito Villarroel, emerged at a time when the city had become increasingly identified as a place of filth and disease, and when Enlightenment ideas of rational reform, education, orderliness and empirical analysis were maintaining that humans had the power to change the environment and reform society, as expressed by Condorcet in his *Esquisse d'un tableau historique des progrès de l'esprit humain* (1795).[3] Given the confidence in man's capacity to alter the environment, and given that the city was increasingly regarded as a dangerous place, the vigilance and regulation of the following elements was believed to be of the utmost importance for public health: air, water, rest and passions, as well as food and drink.

Viceroy Revillagigedo's urban projects for Mexico City were without doubt influenced by two interrelated factors. One was the urban plans and projects proposed by Charles III for Spain, and in particular for Madrid since 1761, and the other was the impact that Enlightenment ideas had on the conception of urban space, when elements such as beauty, symmetry and functionality were of paramount importance.[4] During the reign of Charles III (1759–88), a new style of government was imposed both in Spain and in New Spain, as the Bourbon monarchy began to implement a new set of ideas that corresponded with a critical and rational attitude towards the arts, science, philosophy and the conception of the state. The main objectives of the Bourbon monarchy were to restore the authority of the Crown and to help Spain to regain its former prosperity. To further these ends, the Bourbon monarchy tightened clerical discipline, emphasized its authority over the church, attacked the privileges of the nobility and the guilds, and enacted administrative, fiscal and industrial reforms that were held to be crucial for Mexico City.[5] This new type of government, commonly referred to as Enlightened Despotism, conceived of the state as administrator and regulator whose task was to ensure the well-being of all — or the common or public good — guided by education and orderliness. The aspect I wish to emphasize is that at the time, the idea of good government or *policía* implied the subordination of private or individual interests to those of society as a whole. The Bourbon state justified its unprecedented intervention "by claiming to act in the interest of 'the public', a concept foreign to previous regimes,"[6] and during Revillagigedo's administration, issues relating to public health became fundamental to the Enlightenment ideal of good administration and government.

Public health, which essentially means communal actions taken to avoid disease and other threats to the health and welfare of individuals and the community at large, has been throughout history one of the major preoccupation's of social life.[7] Its areas of concern have included and still include, among others, "the control of transmissible diseases, the control and improvement of the physical environment (sanitation), the provision of water and food in good quality and in sufficient supply, the provision of medical care and the relief of disability and destitution."[8] However, when referring to public health issues, the prevailing medical ideas must not be overlooked, because current notions of medicine have always been a major determining factor in all health policies. When sickness was ascribed to gods or spirits, then prayers, ceremonies and sacrifices were required for healing. When it was believed that most diseases had their origin in and were spread by infested airs — miasmas — that emerged from rotting vegetables, tainted water and human waste, what predominated was the urge to clean the environment, a practice which intensified during times of crisis, such as when epidemics occurred.[9] The association of environmental elements with disease and epidemic outbreaks had by the late eighteenth century a very long tradition, one which dated back to classical writings such as *Airs, Waters, Places* (c. fifth century BC), attributed to Hippocrates and part of the Hippocratic Corpus, and Galen's (AD 126–216) *Hygiene*.[10] The environmental explanation of disease stressed the need to prevent contact with miasmas and to prevent the inhalation of miasmatic exhalations. The word miasma — which derived from the Greek word for stain or pollution — was at the heart of the miasmatic theory of disease, which argued that epidemic outbreaks of infectious diseases were caused by the pathological state of the atmosphere. According to this theory, a particular atmospheric state could "produce certain diseases capable of spreading for the duration of that particular combination of circumstances."[11] In Mexico City, the prevailing medical belief about the origin and spread of disease, in particular epidemic diseases, during the late eighteenth century was that they were the outcome of the infection of the air and water by atmospheric pollution, dirt and filth — or miasmas — but epidemics were also understood as resulting from moral and religious failures.[12] Therefore prayer, special religious processions, quarantines and measures to keep the city clean were the methods used to combat the devastating impact of epidemics.

The stress placed on ordering and cleaning the city during the late eighteenth century assumed a causal relationship between the environment and disease. Because stagnant water and foul odours were regarded as factors responsible for disease, it was thought that they should be removed from populated areas. According to Roy Porter, from the Enlightenment to the mid-nineteenth century, "smell featured crucially in the leading theories of life and disease ... Stench was, in fact, disease."[13] During Revillagigedo's administration, two types of public health measures predominated in Mexico City: emergency measures aimed at restraining the impact of epidemics, and specific measures, laws and regulations concerning the removal of offensive trades and cleaning the city.[14] But the main objective of public health policy was the prevention of epidemics and/or the diminution of their impact. Thus, if the miasmatic exhalations were dispersed by air currents, causing the infection of the air, water and any object in contact with them, the scope of public health policy embraced the entire city.[15] It is therefore not surprising to find that attempts to clean it and clear it of anything that obstructed the free circulation of all elements within it rapidly multiplied. In order to modify the unsanitary conditions of a city, what was required was to introduce specific urban legislation that embraced most social activities, such as the functioning and location of public markets and graveyards, as well as to introduce laws aimed at limiting or ordering the free circulation of people, animals and goods within the city or, as Corbin has stated, "the aim was to develop a fully coherent strategy."[16] Thus, at the same time as this heightened sensitivity to foul odours and sites of accumulation and putrefaction was surfacing, public health became a key to the idea of good administration and government.[17]

Donald Cooper has shown that between 1761 and 1813 Mexico City suffered from the impact of five serious epidemics: in 1761–62 typhus and smallpox; in 1779–80 smallpox; between

1784–87 several epidemic diseases and famine; in 1797–98 smallpox; in 1813 typhus. Among them they claimed at least fifty thousand lives.[18] Cooper has also shown that during the late eighteenth and early nineteenth centuries the practice of medicine was not centred around a particular orthodoxy, and that there was no single predominant way of restoring health. Public health was the concern of different and often competing authorities, and a variety of healing procedures and rituals existed, including magic, prayers, bloodletting, purging, the use of plants and herbs, as well as the attempt to prevent the creation of sites of stagnation.[19]

In Mexico City, public health issues were the concern of the Municipal Council, the Royal Medical Board, established by Royal Decree in 1646,[20] the Viceroy, the High Court and the Church. The Municipal Council was the chief authority, and all its actions had some connection, direct or indirect, with the health and well-being of the citizenry. Three of its main areas of concern were municipal sanitation, water supply and health menaces generated by the inadequate and poorly located cemeteries. The Royal Medical Board was the body responsible for maintaining high professional standards within the medical profession, and examined prospective physicians, surgeons, pharmacists and phlebotomists.[21] It also inspected pharmacies and licensed pharmacists, and was often consulted by the Viceroy in matters relating to medicine and public health. The Church's involvement was very important because of its traditional control of hospitals and cemeteries and because of the spiritual power it exercised over the population. And it was precisely at times of crisis, as when epidemics threatened society, that these diverse authorities worked or attempted to work in a coordinated way, and emergency measures were implemented. The emergency measures included the creation of temporary hospitals, the organization of special religious processions, the allocation of additional funds for food and medicine, lighting bonfires to purify the air, and having the church bells rung at night to reassure the public. In addition, during times of crisis the city was divided into special districts to facilitate the search for people who were sick and to make sure they were placed in emergency or provisional treatment hospitals, or in cemeteries if they had already died.[22]

The Unsanitary City

During the late eighteenth century, the city became increasingly identified as a place of filth and disease, while the rationalism of the Enlightenment perceived the ideal city as organized in accordance with criteria of centrality, symmetry, uniformity and perspective;[23] it should possess specially designated sites for each activity, and its water and air had to be continually moving to prevent the much-feared miasmatic exhalations. Some trades, in particular those that polluted the air and gave off bad odours or miasmas, such as tanneries, had to be removed from populated areas, as did cemeteries, hospitals, public markets and butcher's shops. A city's streets should be wide and adequately paved, its fountains and aqueducts well maintained, and any element within the city that did not contribute to the free circulation of people, goods and/or air had to be modified.[24] The free or unobstructed circulation of all elements within the city would help to diminish the creation of places of stagnation and accumulation. This idea had important implications for both urban planning and public health and was praised as fundamental to the benefit and good government of New Spain.[25]

Many of the directives that guided the urban reforms attempted in Mexico City during the late eighteenth century emerged at a time when the functioning of the city was linked to the functioning of the human body. Emmanuel Le Roy Ladurie has shown that during the course of the eighteenth century a new way of looking at the city emerged in France, a gaze inspired by medicine which imagined the city as having internal organs — a heart, arteries, veins and circulation, as well as excretions.[26] Thus, for the vision of the city-as-organism, the term "functionality" — popularized at the time in the social and political sciences — was of particular importance. In 1770, the term "functionality" was first used in France to refer to the physiology of urban space, and implied that it was essential for the city to possess freedom of movement, or an efficient and unobstructed circulation of all elements within it, be they people, goods, vehicles, air and/or water.[27] And because the city was likened to a human body, it could also suffer from disease, and so it did. A number of urban diseases gained prominence among city observers, and these were not confined to public health issues, but also included questions of social disorder. Thus, poverty, disease, prostitution, overcrowding and air pollution were among the so-called "urban pathologies." For instance, in 1769, Jacques-Vincent Delacroix spoke of the city of Paris as a huge cancer that fed off rural areas; Jean-Jacques Rousseau emphasized the importance of fresh air, simple food and rural simplicity; he viewed cities as unhealthy and stated that "les villes sont le gouffre de l'espèce humaine." And Louis-Sébastien Mercier, in his detailed studies of Paris, the *Tableau de Paris* (ca. 1789), condemned the foul and infectious air the urban population was forced to breathe, the tainted water that ran along the Seine, the adulterated foodstuffs for sale, as well as the dangers posed by cemeteries to the well-being of the urban population.[28]

This new way of looking at the city can be seen in some of the literary representations of Mexico City during the last decades of the eighteenth century. According to Jérôme Monnet, in the numerous chronicles written about the city, from Francisco Cervantes de Salazar's *Segundo Diálogo* of 1554, up to the *Breve Compendiosa Narración de la Ciudad de México* written in 1778 by Juan de Viera, the city had been continually praised for its order and beauty, and the same views on the city had been transmitted from generation to generation, despite epidemics, economic crises, population movements and natural disasters.[29] For more than two centuries, little or nothing had been said in criticism of its unsanitary conditions and its problems. However, during the 1780s, the city ceased to be described as comfortable and beautiful, as an example to follow or as a model in itself. Instead, disorder, foul odours, dirt and anarchy prevailed in a space that for centuries had been described and defined as just the opposite. What took place during the final decades of the eighteenth century was a revolution, and within a very short span of time the inversion of values was complete.[30]

This new perspective on the city can be discerned in the *Discurso sobre la Policía de México; reflexiones y apuntes sobre varios objetos que interesan la salud pública y la policía particular de esta ciudad de México, si se adaptasen las providencias o remedios correspondientes*, written in 1788 by the Regent of the Audiencia, Baltasar Ladrón de Guevara (1726–1804).[31] This work pinpoints and criticizes the city's unsanitary conditions and proposes measures to solve many of its problems, conveying to the reader a model of the ideal city by stressing its negative elements. It is important to note that the *Discurso* was not an isolated work. In 1785, Hipólito Villarroel wrote *Enfermedades políticas que padece la capital de esta Nueva España en casi todos los cuerpos de que se compone y remedios que se la deben aplicar para su curación si se quiere que sea útil al Rey y al público,* and Francisco Sedano wrote *Noticias de México* between 1789 and 1798, leaving an image of the city in which what predominated was filth and stench.[32] The spirit of optimism and the exaltation of the marvels found in the capital of New Spain that had prevailed since the sixteenth century was definitively broken.

The image of the city conveyed by Ladrón de Guevara was dominated by ideas of functionality, systematization of space and good sanitary conditions. The *Discurso* was written both to inspire and to coincide with many of the activities and urban policies dictated by Viceroy Revillagigedo between 1789 and 1794. It was dated 24 November 1788, and covered all aspects of urban life, such as the administration of the city, its public services, the economy and land tenure. One of the main issues it explored was the unsanitary conditions in the city, and it is precisely this aspect that gives coherence to the entire text. Ladrón de Guevara firmly believed that the city had to be thoroughly reorganized, that the result would be beneficial to all the urban population, and that only then would the city have a good government or *policía*. Ladrón de Guevara made detailed studies of the city and he, along with José Antonio de Alzate, was commissioned by Viceroy Martin de Mayorga (1779–83) to make proposals for the improvement of the administration of the capital of New Spain.

Throughout the eighteenth century, attempts were made to reorganize the city into territorial administrative units (as happened in 1713, 1720 and 1750), and in 1782, Guevara's proposal to subdivide the city into eight wards (*cuarteles mayores*) — and each of them into four minor wards (*cuarteles menores*) — was implemented. This reform of urban space meant that the entire city was to be continuously supervised by the newly appointed *alcaldes de barrio,* or ward chiefs. The task of the thirty-two ward chiefs was to assure security, cleanliness and order, to ensure that the people dedicated themselves to their tasks both day and night, and to guarantee that justice was present at all times to prevent vice, apply immediate punishments and maintain good political order.[33] When Ladrón de Guevara explained how he had conceived the idea of dividing the city into territorial administrative units, he said that it had been done on the basis of his knowledge of the city, gained by regularly walking the streets.[34]

The city as described in the *Discurso* must be considered the result of the strong empirical and classificatory tradition of the Enlightenment, and proof of this is that the author carefully analyzed the conditions found in the city's streets and homes; the methods used to dispose of all types of refuse; and the efficiency of the city's sewers, public markets, parks, fountains, abattoirs, among many other sites. He repeatedly stressed the positive impact of the urban reforms experienced in Madrid during the reign of Charles III, and firmly believed that this example could be followed in New Spain. When referring to Madrid, he argued that "from being one the dirtiest [cities] in Europe before Charles III, it is today one of the cleanest."[35] The model of the well-administered and stench-free city looked to the major European cities of the time for guidance and example. Madrid was one of them; other cities named by the author were Venice and London. However, during the 1780s most European cities were far from ordered, but the discourse of the Enlightenment stressed that they should be completely reorganized and their unsanitary conditions improved.[36]

The thorough reorganization and good government of the city was not only important for the economy of Spain and New Spain, but would be in the interest of the common or public good. It was crucial for each activity to have a specific site, and for the urban population to learn to respect the differentiated use of public space. For instance, the widespread practice of selling all sorts of food throughout the city was said to be inappropriate, hindering the free circulation of people and goods, as well as being an insult to the senses of sight and smell. Guevara argued that this practice had to be prohibited and that food should only be allowed to be sold in designated areas.[37] Thus, as in Madrid, the city had to be thoroughly cleansed, its streets cleared of all obstructions, and the urban population discouraged from throwing everything onto communal ground.[38]

The dirtiness of the city was not only viewed as a threat to public health, but also led to an unpleasant perception of the city, causing annoyance to the senses of sight and smell, and giving rise to problems of circulation within the city. Ladrón de Guevara argued that it was important to encourage a change in the day-to-day activities of the population, implying that issues relating to public health had a direct impact on private life. It was not enough to have specific public services, such as an efficient system of waste collection and disposal; the inhabitants had to change their habits and their attitude towards litter and waste, and refrain from littering the streets, canals or public fountains.

Guevara was particularly keen on recommending that streets be adequately paved. Paved streets were not only important in easing the circulation of people and goods within the city; they were also pleasant to look at.[39] Above all, they were a means of sealing off the filth of the soil or the noisomeness of underground water.[40] Another reason why it became increasingly important to have paved streets was that by the mid-eighteenth century many of the lakes within the valley, and indeed the lake that still surrounded parts of the city, Lake Mexico, had suffered from an accelerated process of desiccation due to drainage works. This had led to an increase in the terrestrial circulation of people and goods, and to a growing number of horses and mules in the city. The traditional means of transport — small boats and canoes along the lakes and canals — had become increasingly restricted to limited areas of the city and to specific seasons of the year. The best time of the year to "navigate" within the city was during the rainy season, when the canals had enough water and allowed movement.[41] However, when the inefficient sewers overflowed, or when the water from Lake Texcoco invaded the city, the unpaved streets became rivers of mud, and the miasmas emanating from the environment infected the air, constituting a serious health hazard. Thus water was another key issue explored in the *Discurso*, in particular the foul-smelling water in canals, public fountains and aqueducts. Ladrón de Guevara argued that all canals and public fountains should be kept meticulously clean, and that specific laws be applied to keep them that way throughout the year. Public fountains were one of the main sources of water for the inhabitants, but they were more often than not dirty and smelly, and people used them for all kinds of activities, such as washing clothes, bathing and drinking, regardless of the fact that this water was thought to be a source of disease.[42] The canals (*acequías*) in the city were also sources of great disgust and embarrassment, in particular the *acequía real*, which ran right next to the Palace, the home of the Viceroy.[43] Because it was believed that stagnant courses of water, often clogged with fetid materials, polluted the air and led to putrid fevers, the government, in 1787, "ordered that a large section of the canal in the center of the city be closed to canoe traffic because the stench of these interior canals ... carries a very grave threat of pest."[44]

Ladrón de Guevara was not only concerned about the miasmatic emanations arising from the city's streets, fountains and canals. He also considered the structure of all buildings in the city. All buildings and homes should have a visual consistency or uniformity of style, height and building materials, as well as similar windows and balconies, and should be numbered consecutively and adopt the same typography, as had been done in Madrid, with large, clear and legible numbers.[45] The *Discurso* recommended avoiding constructing tall buildings because they blocked the light from the shorter ones around them, and because they hindered the free circulation of air. Numerous green areas with many trees and plenty of public parks should be built, and as many streets as possible should be lined with trees of equal height.[46] The urban concepts expressed in the *Discurso* emphasized the need to have a linear, symmetrical, uniform and unobstructed city; a city that allowed the free circulation or movement of all elements within it and wherein each activity had a designated site so that proper order and *policía* would benefit everyone.

Ladrón de Guevara's detailed analysis of the city during the last decades of the eighteenth century was not, as mentioned earlier, an isolated work. Hipólito Villarroel, who described himself as "a friend of truth and an enemy of disorder," likened New Spain, in his book *Enfermedades políticas*, to a living body that required a detailed analysis of all of its organs in order to restore it to a healthy condition.[47] Although the author acknowledged that throughout the colonial period there had been numerous attempts to solve many of its problems, they had always failed, and the capital of the New World suffered from a serious pathological state.[48]

Villarroel used medical discourse as an allegorical and moral interpretation of the functioning of New Spain, and the human body became the framework for his analysis of society. By making a detailed analysis of each of its parts, he localized sources of disease in the justice system and in the textile industry, as well as in religious festivals and in the Alameda. Bullfights, the consumption of *pulque* and other alcoholic beverages, the numerous public markets, the tobacco factory and wet-nurses, as well as the Viceroy and the Indians, were thoroughly examined. His dissection of New Spain did not favour the end of Spanish rule; on the contrary, his prescriptions called for a thorough reorganization of the functioning of the colonial authorities, and for the application of force if necessary in the attempt to prevent social disorders. His main objective was to describe solutions which would ensure that all in New Spain would work towards the benefit of the Crown, and not for the fulfillment of self-interest or personal wealth. The King, the Viceroy and the Church were held to be responsible for watching over the diseased state and taking the appropriate measures to root out disorder, the mode of treatment being both moral and physical. He noted that the laws that called for proper administration were not enforced; that the clergy accumulated vast amounts of wealth to the detriment of towns and smaller cities; and that in the city disorder and confusion reigned: "That this capital is only a city because of its name, in reality it is a hamlet, or a mob conformed by an infinite number of peoples where confusion and disorder reign."[49]

Among the remedies that would heal New Spain, Villarroel argued that it was imperative that the dictates of the King were properly followed, and one of the obstacles to this was the great number of issues that continually made demands on the Viceroy, leaving him with neither the time nor the energy to monitor the effectiveness of the edicts and laws. The viceroys, he believed, suffered from "the illness of *Ahitera* or indigestion that is rarely cured; if the patient does not observe a method or if he is not administered a cathartic, the bad humors will not be released."[50] His prescription for purging the waste products that cause disease is a clear appeal to the medical tradition dating from Galen, in the second century AD, that maintained that man was in good health when his body, its parts and humours were in equilibrium, and that one of the methods to restore health was by purging.[51] Villarroel urged the Viceroy to surround himself with competent people capable of dealing with voluminous issues of minor importance (a modern bureaucracy), so that both his time and energy could be fully devoted to the government of New Spain. Another major source of disease was identified in the legal system, described as swollen by a huge number of lawyers who were more concerned with having a comfortable position than with dispensing justice, which should be carried out efficiently, properly and by competent individuals. A phenomenon harshly criticized in *Enfermedades políticas* was the luxurious and ostentatious lifestyle enjoyed by many within the city. Villarroel argued that the yearning of the inhabitants for an unnecessarily luxurious and superfluous lifestyle was the result of the influence of French ideas, and that it had to end.[52]

With regard to the city, Villarroel argued that it was in absolute chaos, it was the "cloaca of the universe," inhabited by an "insolent, barbarous, vice-ridden populace."[53] The filth of the city had it submerged in an "abyss of dirt and ignorance," and its streets and canals "exhale a pestilent stench, harmful to health."[54] Those features were aggravated by the circulation of more than 637 vehicles which caused accidents and deaths, destroyed the pavement (where it existed), and fouled the areas along which they passed. In addition, many vehicles constituted an ostentatious display of wealth and were used with that sole purpose in mind. The numerous laws and edicts that specified that the city had to be cleansed and that all its streets should be paved were not implemented. Those with the responsibility for doing so were never fined or punished for neglecting their duties.

The population of the city, according to Villarroel, was 120,000. Of that figure, he classified forty thousand as parasites and criminals: people with no work, no permanent occupation or home. Most of them, he argued, did not even belong to the city, were from other parts of the colonial domain and came in search of work.[55] The way to free the city from parasites and criminals was to force them to go back to their place of origin, and to build a wall around the city to prevent their future entry. He also thought it was essential to carry out a detailed census of the urban population so that the authorities would know not only how many people lived in the city, but also what occupation they had. Thus it would be possible to identify vagrants.[56] He also argued that the great majority of the urban population led an immoral life, were drunk, behaved like animals and lacked culture and education. He was particularly opposed to the disorders that accompanied the religious celebrations and feast days that proliferated throughout the year, such as Easter, the day of the Dead and the day of the Virgin Mary, and argued that such religious festivities led to all sorts of profanities and immoral actions, to alcoholism and to numerous sins.[57] To alcoholism, in particular the widespread use and abuse of *pulque*, he devoted five sections of the book, urging that it was necessary to extirpate the drunkenness and the "infinite sins and faults that represent an offense to God and to man."[58] The remedies that Villarroel wished to enforce in the city called for a constant supervision of all activities taking place within it; and order, cleanliness and hard work had to be firmly imposed. An efficient and good administration and an urban population that worked, prayed and behaved would guarantee peace, tranquility and harmony among its dwellers, as well as cleanliness throughout the city.[59]

The image of the city that had to be attained was one where order and cleanliness prevailed, a city that would be inhabited by an industrious, law-abiding, religious population, all of whom worked towards the common good of New Spain and respected the authority of the Viceroy and the Church. The city had to cease being the "cloaca of the universe," and the primacy of New Spain regained. Viceroy Revillagigedo's urban proposals attempted to resolve many of the issues set forth by Ladrón de Guevara and by Villarroel. The following section will examine how the proper organization and cleanliness of the city became a key issue in urban administration between 1789 and 1794.

Viceroy Revillagigedo and Urban Sanitation

The Segundo Conde de Revillagigedo arrived as Viceroy to New Spain on 17 October 1789, and aimed to carry out most of the recommendations and proposals that Guevara set forth in his *Discurso*. When he arrived, the city had numerous beautiful buildings and churches, and the concentration and display of wealth in the central district was evident. In addition, it was thought that "the noble and Imperial City of Mexico" could compete with any ancient city of the world, be it "Thebes or Rome."[60] This optimism, which emphasized the city's wealth, architecture, beauty and diversity, was completely contradicted by the writings of both Ladrón de Guevara and Villarroel. Revillagigedo also thought that the city was in need of a thorough overhaul.

However, Viceroy Revillagigedo was neither the first nor the only person to attempt to transform the city during the second half of the eighteenth century. Viceroys Carlos Francisco de Croix (1766–71) and Antonio María de Bucareli y Ursua (1771–79) had also tried to find solutions to many of the city's problems, for example, by protecting the city from the floods that continually threatened it by investing resources in the drainage of Huehuetoca; by adopting a new system for paving the city's streets introduced from France in 1770; and by giving special attention to areas thought to be among the main sources of disease. Viceroy Croix issued in 1769 a "comprehensive edict which addressed itself in great detail to the extremely important object of general cleanliness," and argued that epidemics and other diseases would persist if the inhabitants continued with the practice of dumping everything into the streets, canals and plazas.[61]

When Revillagigedo arrived in New Spain, the city had numerous public works, such as aqueducts and roads, all of vital importance to the health and general well-being of the population, but they were all badly maintained. For instance, the interior drainage system of the city was totally inadequate, and only partial solutions had been found to the chronic threat of floods. In addition, public services, the collection of garbage and refuse and the maintenance of cemeteries were all inadequate, and private sanitary facilities were practically non-existent. "In such an unfavorable physical environment the people were prime targets for the filth-begotten disease such as typhus."[62]

Revillagigedo thought that the recurrent epidemics and the high mortality rates were partly the consequence of the failure of previous administrations to implement good public works and to enforce the laws and regulations enacted to keep the city clean.[63] Revillagigedo was also critical of previous administrators of the city and of the fact that the specific laws were neither respected nor carried out. His wide-ranging activities and concerns with respect to public health and sanitation can be appreciated in the *Instrucción Reservada* he left to his successor, the Marqués de Branciforte,[64] in the *Compendio de providencias de policía del Segundo Conde de Revillagigedo*, and throughout the legislation passed during his administration. In the *Instrucción*, he clearly outlined the specific causes he thought were responsible for epidemics: "the failure to locate cemeteries safely beyond populated areas," — (indeed, many corpses were inadequately buried at the entrance of the Cathedral and inside churches);[65] "the reuse of clothing that had been taken from the sick and the dead" (as second-hand clothes were sold or given to the poor); "the unrestrained wanderings of cows, hogs, and other animals, through the streets of the city, the practice of the poor of going about naked, or nearly so, and the scant respect for hygiene both in public places and in private homes."[66] In the face of such a chaotic situation, Revillagigedo's recommendations were extraordinarily wide-ranging, and included the cleansing and paving of streets and plazas; illuminating dark and dangerous areas; reorganizing the police force; building gardens and parks; extending the supply of water; and draining all areas saturated with water, as well as organizing an efficient system of waste collection and disposal, among many other issues.[67] It was also during Revillagigedo's administration that the first population census of Mexico City and of New Spain was carried out, representing a clear response to the empirical tradition of the Enlightenment. The *Censo de Revillagigedo,* as it is now known, established that for the year 1790–91 the city had 112,926 inhabitants.[68]

Revillagigedo attempted to establish permanent measures that would keep the city in a satisfactory sanitary condition at all times, and not only during periods of epidemic. This was because matters relating to public health were taken to be related to the larger political issue of good government. For instance, in 1790, Revillagigedo issued a law made up of fourteen sections. Each section detailed the obligations, rights, restrictions and time by which each person responsible for cleaning the city was bound. It also established fixed days and hours for the collection of litter and disposal of human waste by special vehicles commissioned for this purpose.[69] All homes had to have cesspools (*común*), so that at night, the special vehicles could also clear them. In order to avoid their stagnation and the resulting miasmas, it was forbidden to foul the water of the canals that ran through various parts of the city. The inhabitants of the city not only had to comply with the dictates of urban hygiene or sanitary reform, but were also subject to a law which prohibited them from being in specific areas of the city unless fully dressed.[70]

The emphasis was on making the city a functional space, in that public space had traditionally been — and still was — a site where many different activities took place simultaneously. For instance, during Revillagigedo's administration, public markets ceased to be unregulated, and some were placed for the first time in specific designated areas. According to Francisco Sedano, the Plaza Mayor before Revillagigedo's administration had been occupied by a public market and butchers' shops, and there had been a cemetery at the entrance to the Cathedral. The Plaza Mayor was completely disorganized, full of street vendors, litter, mud, with no order whatsoever.[71] Taking advantage of the festivities that took place in 1789, from 27 to 28 December, to commemorate the beginning of the reign of Charles IV, Viceroy Revillagigedo ordered that the Plaza Mayor be cleared of all commerce and people, as was usual during important celebrations. However, a law was then issued which stated that none of the previous activities would be allowed back in that space.

All commercial activities were relocated to the purposely-built market in the Plaza del Factor and to the market of the Plaza del Volador, the fountain and gallows disappeared, and the ground was completely paved.[72]

What was attempted during the final years of the eighteenth century was the creation of an unobstructed circulation of air, people and goods in the city. Only when this free circulation was achieved would the city become a beautiful and comfortable site and benefit the public good and public order. What was attempted was to create an urban environment that would display the rational organization of public space, and to imbue the poor with new habits of tidiness and industry.[73] A central feature of the urban renovation campaigns was cleanliness. However, it is important to point out that during the course of the final decades of the eighteenth century, cleanliness referred not only to the removal of dirt. Cleanliness was above all related to movement and the avoidance of stagnation.[74] A clean city was one that allowed its water and air to circulate freely, and the movement of these elements was regarded as crucial in the struggle against disease. Therefore, areas where there was an accumulation of litter, waste, water and/or decomposing matter were considered sources of miasmas, and hence of disease and, in the worst cases, of epidemics. The primary goal was to ensure the evacuation of rubbish.[75] And just as public markets became identified as possible agents of disease unless adequately supervised and organized, stagnant water within the city, be it that of canals, aqueducts, fountains, sewers or that of Lake Texcoco, became identified as real threats to the good order and policy of New Spain, and as issues of public health. The objective was to ensure that all water was in continuous movement, to avoid the creation of marshes and swamps, and to take all tainted water and litter out of and far from populated areas.

Revillagigedo's ideas for ordering the city and thus allowing an unobstructed circulation of all elements within it were crucial in terms of public health and the prevailing notions about the causes of disease, but also with respect to the aesthetic appearance of the city. The convergence of these issues can be seen in the 1794 map of the city drawn by the master builder of the city, architect Ignacio Castera, the *Plano ignográfico de la ciudad de México que demuestra el reglamento general de sus calles, así para la comodidad y hermosura, como para la corrección y extirpación de las maldades que hay en sus barrios, por la infinidad de sitios escondidos, callejones sin tránsito, ruinas de paredones ...*, It was defined by Francisco de la Maza as the first attempt to organize the future growth of the city, as well as representing the emergence of modern urbanism in Mexico.[76] This map emphasized the lengthening and straightening of streets that, it was hoped, would cross the entire city, from the Plaza Mayor to the edges or indigenous wards. Long and unobstructed streets would allow the circulation of people, goods and air as well as the construction of consecutively numbered houses and buildings. The map also delineated the sites where public works such as pavements, aqueducts, canals and underground pipelines had to be built, what direction they had to take and what had been achieved up to that point.

The city was envisaged with a perfectly symmetrical square layout, with four plazas at each extreme, all having the same dimensions and distance between them. Beyond the plazas, the entire city was to be surrounded by an open ditch, or *Acequía Maestra*, whose purpose would be to collect rainwater, and water from the interior canals and the sewers. The aesthetic ideas of Castera's project corresponded to an urban concept dominated by the ideas of symmetry, straight lines and movement. Thus, issues relating to aesthetic sensitivity and public health converged. However, despite the efforts and plans for the city during the late eighteenth century, the urban reforms supported by Revillagigedo enjoyed only partial success, and he faced considerable opposition to many of his plans due to the financial costs involved, and owing to the ideological imposition they represented.

After the end of Revillagigedos's term in office, on 9 January 1795, Mexico City's Municipal Council issued a formal complaint against him, and he was charged with offences that included "having improperly ordered the arrangement of the city markets, naming the streets and numbering the houses, and of establishing various new public fountains."[77] He was also found responsible for the inadequacy of the sewage system built during his administration, which according to the Municipal Council led to the floods of 1793 and 1794, but the Council of Indies declared that all the charges against Revillagigedo were untrue.[78] However, it must be stressed that the significance of the numerous laws, projects and proposals introduced during the government of Revillagigedo rests on the influence they had on subsequent Mexico City administrations well into the nineteenth century.[79] This can be seen throughout the nineteenth century, when he was continuously named and remembered as the "best" viceroy New Spain had ever had. Also, during the mid-nineteenth century, it was widely believed that the most important and transcendental proposals for the city, in particular those that were directly related to public health, had been those of the late eighteenth century.[80] The proposal to build a statue of Revillagigedo in 1868 to commemorate his works for the city also reflects this view, and one of the major objectives embraced by the Porfirian administration a hundred years after Revillagigedo was to transform the city into a well-organized, hygienic and prosperous world capital.

Although in the late nineteenth century the idea of transforming the physical environment was a crucial component of Mexico City's urban policy, and although it was no longer the Enlightenment idea of the public good or of good government and administration which guided the reforms, many of the objectives set down during the late eighteenth century were only accomplished during the final decades of the nineteenth century.

After Mexico's independence from Spain in 1821, the new nation's lack of economic and political stability hampered the enactment of comprehensive and far-reaching policies.[81] Public health policies remained limited to ad hoc municipal measures in response to emergencies, and long-term institutional development was sporadic and ineffective. Furthermore, many measures implemented during the late eighteenth century were reinforced — by either liberals or conservatives — well into the nineteenth century.[82] For instance, in 1824, José Mendívil, governor of the Federal District, issued a *Bando de policía y buen gobierno* that was more than reminiscent of the sanitary dispositions of Revillagigedo. This law placed particular emphasis on establishing penalties to sanction anyone found to be fouling public areas, fountains, aqueducts, and any other site, while men and women were ordered to maintain in good order the fronts of their houses and were prohibited from selling food and clothes in the city's streets.[83] However, those measures proved inefficient when Asiatic cholera reached Mexico through the port of Tampico in 1833, a date that was particularly critical for the new nation. [84] The country was in the midst of political upheavals and armed conflicts that emanated from the liberal reforms that Vice-President Valentín Gomez Farías and the radical deputies to the national Congress attempted to introduce with the aim of transforming the relationship between church and state. And while conservatives and the Church blamed the liberal reforms for the appearance of cholera, fourteen thousand people died in Mexico City due to the epidemic outbreak.[85] The tensions and conflicts between central state intervention and federal autonomy, and those that emerged between the liberal reformers, conservatives and the power and influence of the Church in matters relative to the control of burying grounds, hospitals and health policies, remained largely unresolved until the late 1860s.[86]

However, it was precisely during the cholera years[87] that the concepts of labour, disease and dirt began to have interchangeable meanings, and when an intolerance towards dirt led European social theorists to fashion a "religion of hygiene." [88] A country capable of equipping itself against epidemics had to rely on social and individual hygiene, and sanitary reform and hygienic education gradually became two of the most important political obligations of the state.

The disastrous consequences for human life and to international commerce that followed upon the cholera epidemics prompted European nations to hold the first Sanitary Conference in 1851.[89] Paris hosted the first of ten such conferences that took place during the course of the nineteenth century, and public health, hygiene and sanitation became increasingly presented as indispensable requirements for protecting the people against their own imprudence and as crucial for the progress and civilization of a nation. In those international settings, diverse physicians, administrators, politicians and industrialists of both Europe and the American continent emphasized that all countries should adopt a general sanitary administration, and that international organization and co-operation was paramount to the advance of science, to commerce and to health.

Although it was only during the final decades of the nineteenth century that the first comprehensive health policy was established and directed by the Mexican state, during the 1830s and 1840s important developments prefigured the more interventionist role that the state was to adopt in health issues. Medical education, research and the practice of medicine became increasingly state-regulated as of 1831, when the Royal Medical Board was suppressed by president and physician Anastasio Bustamante, and its place occupied by the Medical Faculty of the Federal District (Facultad Médica del Distrito Federal). Three years later, the Medical Science Establishment (Establecimiento de

Ciencias Médicas) was created with the exclusive right to oversee medical education and public sanitation.[90] In addition, medical associations and societies flourished from the 1830s onwards, and medical and scientific journals appeared, wherein the most important breakthroughs in the medical sciences were made public.[91] However, the most far-reaching law for the purpose of medical study and for public health policy was issued in 1841.[92]

On 4 January of that year, the Superior Sanitation Council of the Department of Mexico was created, all of whose members were directly appointed by the government. Its obligations included the supervision of medical education and the practice of medicine, and it was to work with the Municipal Council in all matters relative to public health and sanitation.[93] But above all, it had the task of creating a Sanitary Code. Nonetheless, the constant climate of political instability, the scant resources destined for medical education, research and public health, and the foreign interventions to which the country was subject, rendered this task impossible until 1891.

By the late nineteenth century, public health was regarded as an indispensable requirement for the material progress of all nations, and important breakthroughs in the medical sciences had gradually led to a new understanding of the origin and prevention of disease and to the acceptance of the germ theory of disease causation. In Mexico, as in other countries, the new scientific information on the germ theory did not immediately displace older notions of disease causation. It took much discussion, controversy and deliberation before the germ theory of disease ascended to the privileged status of a "scientific truth," and Mexican physicians and public health officials during the Porfiriato considered a thorough sanitary reform to be essential.

By the late 1870s, public health had become an institutionalized branch of government, and the state's involvement was not limited to times of crisis. Mexico City had become the centre of education and research facilities as well as the focal point of research undertaken by public health officials, engineers, architects, land surveyors, and in particular of work carried out by the Superior Sanitation Council. As dirt, stagnant water, inadequate sewers and disease were identified, solutions were recommended, and sometimes effective action followed.

The threats posed to public health during the Porfiriato were identified in two areas in particular, one being the environment, and the other being society. The environmental threats were located in the city's inefficient drainage system, which led to regular flooding, stagnant water and bad odours, and in the use of Lake Texcoco as the final destination of all the city's sewage. The social threat was pinned on the urban poor, and it was held that because they were filthy and poor they could cause disease. Public health officials believed there was a connection between the moral and the material. If material improvements were efficiently carried out — and they were there to make sure this was the case — then the standards of living would improve. What was also required was to teach the poor the principles of public and private hygiene, which involved moral reform. Public health officials often explained society as a "social organism," and argued that the only possible way of studying it was through the application of scientific principles. These scientific principles included a common methodological approach, observation, classification, and more observation and statistics, as well as experts from different disciplines. Through the objectivity and unquestionable truth of quantitative data and of scientifically structured observations, public health officials and the state, it was believed, would possess the empirical basis for both policies and programs.

Physicians and hygienists embarked on detailed studies of the city and advised on reforms, and the capital became the core of the scientific investigation of society. Some of the solutions proposed included the construction of an adequate drainage system and cleansing the city of all that fouled the air, corrupted the water and tarnished the image of public places, as well as making sure that the urban poor learned the principles of hygiene, be it by education or by force. Public health officials embarked on a range of activities, one of their goals being the scientific progress of the nation. The next chapter will examine why the city's environment was regarded as a threat to health, what arguments were advanced and what measures were proposed to alter the environment. This task was to absorb the attention of the government, physicians, engineers, architects and public health officials.

2

The Control of the Environment

The Community of Hygienists

Physicians and hygienists were greatly concerned with the state of public health in Mexico City, and firmly believed they could contribute to the progress of the country. Their contribution or mission was twofold. First, through the application of their sanitary and hygienic knowledge, essential to urban design and planning, the city could be regenerated; and second, through the teaching or inculcation of the principles of private and public hygiene, the habits of the urban population would be transformed. The city would cease to be a dirty, foul-smelling, disorganized place, and would possess numerous parks, adequately drained and paved streets and efficient public works. And the urban population, through education, hygiene — and force, if necessary — would cease to be ignorant, superstitious, vice-ridden and infectious. Only when these things were achieved would the capital be able to display proudly the advancement of the nation as appropriate to the era of order and progress made possible by the Porfirio Díaz government.

The concerns of hygienists were so broad that delimiting them with a precise boundary is difficult. Their areas of interest included working class housing, schools, hospitals, public markets, gardens, parks and plazas, cemeteries, sewers, stagnant waters, abattoirs, factories and any other site that could have a detrimental effect on public health. Because illness could be caused by almost anything, everything had to be considered.

This meant that their program as hygienists was all-embracing, and that they needed to have confidence in their methods for detecting, deciphering and proposing measures to transform the environment. These methods included detailed observations, scientific inquiries, chemical and meteorological analyses, topographical surveys, statistics, case studies and personal communications, among others. Hygienists created a discourse that encompassed society as a whole; they forged close links between the notions of order, cleanliness and hygiene, and in their practice made little distinction between them.[1]

Most hygienists studied medicine. In Mexico City, it was taught at the National School of Medicine (Escuela Nacional de Medicina), at the Armed Forces Medical School (Escuela Práctica Médico-Militar) and at the Armed Forces College (Colegio Militar), and what distinguished them from other physicians was that they were devoted to public service. Although some worked in hospitals, many were employed by the Superior Sanitation Council, the Ministry of Economic Development, the Municipal Council or other government institutions, and some were self-employed. However, not all hygienists or public health officials emerged from the medical profession; some were engineers (sanitary engineers in particular), and others were architects, although at the time there was not such a clear-cut distinction between architecture and engineering as there is today.

During the initial years of the Porfiriato, the National School of Medicine had 126 students, 17 professors and 10 teaching assistants. By 1899, the number of students had risen to 373, and the number of teaching assistants to 60. By 1900, 42 architects, 82 dentists, 307 pharmacists, 884 engineers and 526 doctors practised their professions in the Federal District and in Mexico City. These professionals were the intellectual elite of the Porfirian regime.[2] Even though they represented different educational backgrounds, methods and objectives, when their gaze was focused upon the unsanitary conditions that prevailed in the city, their ideas converged. They aimed to show that their knowledge of society and of the threats posed to the city by the environment and the lack of hygienic practices among the population was scientifically and morally valid. They relied upon a number of ways of upholding their claims. Two of them were of particular importance: their use of statistical information, and their first-hand observations or diagnoses of the city. However, before dealing with the authority that statistical information bestowed upon physicians, hygienists and other public health officials, it is important to emphasize briefly the importance of science and the scientific method for the implementation of hygienic, sanitary and public health programs.

Charles Hale has shown that the political consensus of late-nineteenth-century liberalism in Mexico was upheld by a set of philosophical ideas that proclaimed the triumph of science. This set of ideas, commonly referred to as positivism, lacks an accepted definition, but as Hale points out, positivism in its philosophical sense is a theory of knowledge in which the scientific method represents man's only means of knowing. Its methods are observation, experimentation and the search for the laws of phenomena or the relationships between them.[3] As a set of social ideas, positivism argued that society was a developing organism, not a collection of individuals, and that the only effective way of studying society was through history.[4] The key to the scientific management of the society was to develop an elite that could provide the leadership for social regeneration. Thus, a strong government — embodied in Porfirio Díaz — was essential. "Weak governments are the sure symptoms of death," Justo Sierra stated in 1880, and a more forthright and clear appeal to authoritarianism was spelled out by Francisco G. Cosmes in 1878:

> Rights! Society now rejects them. What it wants is bread ... a little less of rights in exchange for a little more of security, order, and peace. We have already enacted innumerable rights, which produce only distress and malaise in society. Now let us try a little tyranny, but honorable tyranny, and see what result it brings.[5]

The advocates of scientific politics, as Hale has shown, called for a strong government, including constitutional reform to lengthen the presidential term as well as to strengthen administrative power. These ideas came into conflict with the classical liberal ideas of constitutional law and individual rights. However, what must be stressed is that science and the scientific method were held to be crucial for the investigation of the society, and that all policies had to be formulated scientifically.

Physicians and hygienists were of the opinion that transforming the city and its inhabitants required a thorough scientific diagnosis; only then could the solutions be applied. These thorough studies of society required research, organization, administration and an increasing bureaucratization for the gathering and analysis of quantitative data, and became a key component of the practice of public health officials within the city.

The Contradictory Proofs of Progress and the City

During the Porfiriato, statistics gained acceptance as undeniable evidence of the modernization of the country. The figures indicating national growth, industrial establishments, railways and mines, among others, all showed that national growth and prosperity were indeed rising.[6] Progress was a cumulative process, and another proof of this modernization was that the population of the country was increasing, in particular the number of people who lived in the capital, the centre of attention of most national and foreign investors, and the focus of public health officials. In 1858, the estimates placed Mexico City's population at around two hundred thousand; in 1895 the figure had risen to 329,774; in 1900 to 344,721, and by 1910 it had grown to 471,066.[7] Population growth was primarily caused by internal migration. A high proportion of migrants could be found in the states of Quintana Roo and Coahuila, but the Federal District and Mexico City received more than a quarter of the total number of migrants between 1895 and 1910. In 1895, a total of 87,379 people from other states arrived in the capital; by 1900, the figure had risen to 151,037, and in 1910, 142,169 people settled in the city. Most of them had come from the states of Guanajuato, Querétaro, Jalisco, Michoacán and Veracruz, often in search of better living and working conditions.[8] As the population of the capital increased, Miguel Macedo explained the rural-urban migration as being the result of the insuperable attraction of the comfort and pleasures life in big cities had to offer. However, the country had few comfortable or pleasurable cities. By 1910, the country had 15,160,377 inhabitants, seventy-one per cent of whom lived in rural areas.[9] However, statistics also showed less pleasurable images of progress. In 1880, doctor Agustín Reyes presented a statistical report to the Superior Sanitation Council in which he stated that the average lifespan for the capital's population during 1878 was 25.5 years. He added that in Paris the average lifespan had amounted to 46.6 years in 1876, almost twice that of Mexico City in 1879.[10]

Premature death and disease shocked the Porfirian public health officials. In 1900, the infant mortality rate was 392 per thousand live births; the annual mortality rate was 33.6 per thousand people, and the average life expectancy of Mexicans was only 26.5 years.[11] These figures gave rise to concern, which was expressed in most scientific publications and newspaper editorials. In 1877, for instance, the scientific and technical journal *El Mundo Científico*, described as a "serious weekly devoted to the popularization of the sciences" and directed by Santiago Sierra, published several articles by Justo Sierra in which he argued that the unsanitary conditions in the capital required a prompt solution and noted official indifference to the possibility of a typhus epidemic.[12] Thus, statistical information also provided a contradictory image of progress; the population was increasing, national production rising, railroads eased national and international commercial activities and population movements; foreign investments and national resources increased industrial output, but the capital of the country had one of the highest mortality rates in the world, and disease and filth threatened the progress of the nation.

Physicians, and in particular hygienists, attempted to reconcile the contradictory images of progress. One of the methods used was to create a linguistic barrier that separated those who had the knowledge and the scientific authority to inspect the city and recommend solutions to urban health problems from those who did not, implying that hygienists were the interpreters of the grand narrative of progress. Another of their methods involved advertising the benefits that would be delivered through the construction of public works essential for urban sanitation. Public works were seen as material evidence of the advances achieved by the country, which would have a trickle-down effect on the urban population. At the same time, statistical information became a crucial factor in establishing the legitimacy of public health officials' opinions and recommendations.

The gathering of statistical information and the ability of the government to compile statistics were regarded as results of the era of social peace that prevailed after decades of political struggles, civil wars and foreign interventions. The General Board of Statistics (Dirección General de Estadística), created on 26 May 1882, was charged with the gathering, classification and publication of all available data about the country.[13] However, since 1872 the use of statistics and of scientifically structured observations had been regarded as crucial for solving urban health problems. In that year, the Ministry of the Interior had ordered the Superior Sanitation Council to collate and submit statistical information on the city, with the aim of establishing medical statistics for the Federal District.[14] Thus, ten years before the creation of the General Board of Statistics, physicians acknowledged that statistics were one of the tools in their struggle against the propagation of disease. This was the first time that statistical information was systematically gathered and analyzed by them. After 1882, the main publishers and users of statistics were the General Board of Statistics, the Mexican Society of Geography and Statistics and the Superior Sanitation Council.[15]

The first three national censuses also took place during the Porfiriato, in 1895, 1900 and 1910, and on all three occasions the results were criticized, the methods questioned, and a general skepticism prevailed when the demographic figures were made public. It is important to note that at least two important public figures greatly concerned about health issues in Mexico City had a direct involvement in the gathering and publishing of statistics. One of them was Dr. Eduardo Liceaga, president of the Superior Sanitation Council from 1886 to 1914. In 1890, Liceaga suggested to General Porfirio Díaz that the Mexican Society of Geography and Statistics should help the Superior Sanitation Council to carry out a census of the population of the capital. The objective was to have precise figures on the number of premature deaths. When the figures became known, they indicated that the population of the city was 324,365; the expected figure was 450,000.[16] The disappointment could not have been greater. The other public figure was physician and historian Antonio Peñafiel, who became one of the most committed public health experts in matters related to the availability and distribution of drinking water, and it was he who prepared all three national censuses.[17]

It is important to stress that the use of statistical information by late-nineteenth-century public health officials in Mexico City legitimized their practices as scientific and valid. Statistics influenced readers because numbers were regarded as objective, scientifically structured, neutral data; they were thought to reveal the links in a given society between its mortality rates and the prevailing diseases, and their use made any argument more convincing. Thus, statistics both helped to legitimize the readings physicians, hygienists and other public health officials took of the city, and at the same time shaped the government's perception of the capital. The use of statistical data by public health officials led to the development of public health as a science of urban society, and the gathering of quantitative data provided an empirical basis for the development and implementation of both policies and programs.[18]

In the opinion of one of the most important hygienists of late nineteenth century Mexico, Dr. Luis E. Ruiz, demography was the collective description of the humane race via statistics, and statistics were nothing other than the accountability of hygiene.[19] For him, as for other hygienists, statistical information was one of the pillars of hygiene, and its methods of investigation were absolutely scientific:

> The essential bases of hygiene as in other fields of knowledge, has gone through three different theoretical stages: theological, metaphysical and scientific … it has followed the progressive development of the human spirit as a whole.[20]

Statistical information, as the previous statement shows, was one of the methods used by public health officials to analyze society and to support their claims, and although statistics possessed neither methodological consistency, nor continuity, they were generally supplemented by personal observations that provided them with the specificity they often lacked.[21] The use and perception of statistical information as scientific, objective and valid for understanding public health problems was one of the characteristics of the sanitary or public health movement of the nineteenth century.[22]

During and after the arrival of cholera in Europe and North and South America in the 1830s, the public health or sanitary movement acquired particular vigour and was inextricably linked to the changing role of the state in transition to industrial society.[23] The public health or sanitary movement attempted to respond to the consequences of the processes of industrialization and increased urbanization in a number of countries, notably in England. The movement postulated that the connection between the environment and disease involved new methods of analysis. In particular, it stressed that social statistics had the power to elucidate the causes of disease within a community and to provide the factual basis for social action. This led sanitary reformers to continue with their inspections and surveys, while statistics became the new tools for demonstrating "the extent to which urban, industrial society created its own special health problems."[24] However, it should be stressed that statistics and surveys could tell different interpreters different things. While some could be drawn to conclude from the data analyzed that the miasmatic influences were responsible for disease, others could express the view that in reality it was the ignorance, backwardness and immorality of the urban population — in particular the urban poor — that led to disease and premature death. The topographical and social analysis of the spread of disease and epidemics "revealed links between poverty, overcrowding and lack of sanitation,"[25] and radical reforms were thought as essential for the survival in and of cities.

According to Ann F. La Berge, the application of statistics to medical and public health issues became important because hygienists used statistics to consolidate theories that there was a concomitance between the advance of civilization and the progress of public health. In addition, statistical analyses furnished scientific proof that this theory was correct; statistics were also used to measure the effect of public health reform and to answer health questions about the causes of disease and mortality.[26]

Mexican physicians, hygienists and the governing elite agreed that the advance of civilization and the progress of public health went hand in hand. Statistics were seen as a science that unveiled facts, but these facts were far from being undisputed or apolitical. The capacity to gather, publish and use statistics during the Díaz regime required the centralization of national power. Through them, attempts were made to impose order on most social and economic activities. To quantify people, properties, activities, births and deaths became not only a requirement for science, knowledge and the administration of the country, but also symbolized the presence and authority of the state throughout the country.[27]

Thus, during the Porfiriato, statistical information became a key component of public health officials assumptions about the causes of premature death and disease, and of the understanding and attempts to find a definitive solution to many of the city's problems. Through the use of statistical information, both national and foreign, public health officials aimed to confirm and reinforce their ideas about the causes of the unsanitary conditions in the city. They identified, defined and illustrated disease and contamination, and relied upon statistics when they claimed that it was imperative to transform the city and its environment. However, there was one issue that did not require statistics in order to be identified as a latent threat. This was the city's natural environment. In order for the city to be able to display the progress achieved by the country, it was imperative to control the menacing aspects of the environment — to control nature and civilize it.

Dangerous Elements

Most studies, analyses, newspaper articles and editorials written in Mexico City about the capital had something to say about the negative impact of the surrounding environment on public health. The most menacing threats were the proximity of Lake Texcoco and the inadequate sewers in the city. Both were believed to poison the atmosphere, contaminate water and cause disease. For centuries, Lake Texcoco had been used as a receptacle for all the city's refuse, and there had been numerous attempts to rid the city of the invasion of tainted water.

Thus, a major concern for public health officials was precisely the threat Lake Texcoco represented to the city, and the questions frequently asked by engineers, state agencies and hygienists were: What should be done with the lake? Should it be drained? Cleansed? And, how would any measure adopted affect public health? According to Dr. José Güijosa, Lake Texcoco served as a receptacle of all the city's refuse, its emanations contaminated the city's atmosphere, and the medical constitution of the capital was seriously altered by this marsh.[28]

Engineers, physicians and state agencies all knew that because of the geographical location of the city, the capital had suffered from numerous floods since its foundation by the Aztecs, and that all the attempts to prevent water taking over parts of the city had failed. During the Porfiriato, public health officials and state agencies, as well as national and foreign capital, brought together their expertise and knowledge and aimed to make the city a safe and modern one. This implied that the intellectual, scientific and financial elites of the Porfirio Díaz regime buried their differences and jealousies to "promote, secularize, medicalize and diffuse water."[29]

The idea that held that the control of the untamed environment surrounding and threatening the city was in itself a civilizing mission can be seen in a speech delivered by Senator Genaro Raigosa in 1881. On 16 November, Raigosa addressed the Chamber of Senators with the aim of portraying the harmful effect that the environment had on the capital and its inhabitants.[30] As was common at the time — and no serious study would embark upon explaining the city's situation without presenting a historicist approach to the problems it had faced since its foundation by the Aztecs — Raigosa argued that the legacy of three hundred years of Spanish domination had been the destruction of the rich vegetation of the valley and city of

Mexico. What remained was a sterile, arid and dusty environment that harmed the atmosphere, altered the climate, polluted the water, and contaminated everything in the city. His appeal to a foundational past, to an ancient and almost mythical origin wherein pure water, prosperity and civilization had reigned, contrasted sharply with the situation he and his contemporaries were confronted with.[31]

Raigosa was of the opinion that if the valley and city of Mexico had once enjoyed the benefits and health-giving elements of a rich, diverse and exuberant vegetation, of clean and odourless lakes and canals, and if it had once been inhabited by a vigorous and healthy population, the situation by the 1880s was completely different. The entire region was inhabited by a miserable populace who succumbed to premature death and disease. The city, the centre of civilization and culture, was surrounded by an unmanageable environment that threatened the health of the capital. Raigosa, by appealing to the notions of health and prosperity, excluded political divisions, discussions and differences from his speech, and aimed to unite the country against a common enemy: the unsanitary conditions that prevailed in its capital. And one of the main problems directly linked to the geographical location of the city was that the ground below the surface of the capital was saturated with water because the city had expanded onto terrain that had once been covered by a system of lakes.

When the city of Mexico-Tenochtitlán was founded in 1325, it was built on a small area of insular marshland within a huge lake system that extended over an estimated area of 1,575 square kilometres. The lake system was located at the central and lowest part of the valley of Mexico[32] and was fed by numerous water sources found within the valley and by various rivers, especially the Cuautitlán, Avenida de Pachuca, Magdalena, Tenango and Tlalmanalco. The area occupied by the lakes decreased rapidly after 1524, when the Spaniards began to rebuild the city after its destruction during the Conquest. By 1861, only 230 square kilometres remained, and in 1891 this had decreased to 95 square kilometres. The only lakes that remained within the area occupied by the city during the Porfiriato were fractions of Lakes Chalco, Texcoco and Xochimilco.[33] In 1881, although the lakes had by then diminished considerably in size, Senator Raigosa explained that it was only necessary to dig eighty centimetres below the surface of the city to find the hidden lake.

This underground lake was a menace to everyone and everything in the city. Its water was rich in saltpetre, organic waste, fecal materials and all sorts of refuse, and increased the porosity of the city's soil, particularly in the east and northeast. In addition, the soil's humidity and capacity for retaining water were elements that posed threats to the population, as well as to the buildings, whose structures lacked a solid and firm foundation and could collapse. Raigosa considered that many buildings were not only on the brink of collapse, but also that they had

> the repugnant appearance of lepers. First they lose part of their skin and little by little they see their body go to pieces. And unless continuous and expensive repair is undertaken, it will not be long before they suddenly collapse due to the lack of support in their destroyed foundations.[34]

The underground water was continuously fed by rainfall, by the swamps surrounding the city and by Lake Texcoco, and it destroyed the remaining vegetation in the capital, causing most of its public gardens to appear to be arid and sterile.[35] Raigosa considered that the loss of the city's vegetation had additional negative consequences for the inhabitants of the capital. In his opinion, before the Spanish Conquest the city had been covered and surrounded by green areas; however, New Spain had been built through the destruction of the valley's vegetation, leading to an insufficient supply of oxygen for its inhabitants.[36] Thus, because of the lack of trees and plants, the atmosphere had been altered, and the once greatly cherished climate of the city transformed. He added that the sudden and drastic changes of temperature, and the lack of humidity, increased the incidence of pneumonia and anemia, degenerated the Mexican race, and produced feeble and weak individuals "with no moral energy or physical vigor."[37] According to the Senator, both anemia and pneumonia were linked to the atmospheric conditions, but anemia was also caused by the loss of nutrients in the vegetation due to the impact of deforestation. The shortcomings of a diseased population meant that the Mexican race would become weaker, both physically and morally. Thus, control of the environment was essential not only for the city but also for the future of the country — its inhabitants. In addition, the environment was considered to encourage crime, and violent crimes were singled out as contributing to the high incidence of premature death in the city. The criminologist Julio Guerrero affirmed that the widespread malaise in the capital, namely crime and vice, was worsened by violent climatic changes and atmospheric alterations brought about by the lack of vegetation.[38]

However, the most dangerous source of disease, as has been mentioned, was Lake Texcoco. It must be stressed that throughout the colonial period this lake had been identified as one of the main sources of disease, and that during the sixteenth century the entire lake system, of which Lake Texcoco was part, had been held to possess mysterious properties, and had been associated with the devil and the Beast described by St. John in the Apocalypse.[39] By the late nineteenth century, Lake Texcoco had lost that eschatological association, but it continued to be associated with more modern and secular evils: damage to the health and hygiene of the Mexican people and to the future of the nation. Water both within the city and in Lake Texcoco, was regarded as a negative element that should either be eradicated or freely circulated. It was imperative to avoid the stagnation of water and the creation of marshes or swamps. However, the constant inspections of the waters in the city made reference to their swamp-like condition and underlined the terrible odours and miasmas that emerged from them, causing disease. The putrefying water that could at any time come to the surface did not need to be seen: it could be smelled. Due to the threat that this huge cesspool posed to the city, there were numerous scientific expeditions to the lake in order to carry out analyses. One of them took place in 1883.

On 11 March 1883, Dr. Antonio Peñafiel and a group of other physicians made a detailed inspection of Lake Texcoco to assess with their own eyes (and, it could be added, also with their noses) the effect that this marsh had on the city. It was thought that March was a favourable month in which to undertake the inspection because the rainy season had not begun. Therefore they would be able to analyze both the water and the land due to the lake's shallowness. Because it was inconvenient to reach the lake by water, that is, by traveling along the Canal de San Lázaro, which discharged all the city's refuse into the lake, they decided that it would be better to make the journey on foot, alongside the canal. This approach would also allow them to see the impact of the salt water of the lake on the surrounding environment and on the living organisms in the lake. As they approached it, the stench became stronger, leading them to question their decision to continue. At the exact point where the Canal de San Lázaro merged with the lake, the vegetation became more sparse, the edges of the lake were dry and displayed a huge cemetery of dead molluscs and insects that burned in the heat and gave off a terrible stench, similar to that which emanates from rotting seafood.[40] This stench, according to Dr. Peñafiel, was more and more frequent in the capital, and was harmful to the health of anyone who came into contact with its putrid emanations. Among the stenches considered particularly dangerous to health were those that arose from areas of stagnation and accumulation, and Peñafiel considered that the threat posed by the stagnant lake water, and by the emanations that emerged from it and reached the city on the prevailing air currents, was nothing other than the complete suffocation of the capital.[41]

The doctors were able to observe the geographical location of the lake in relation to the city, and its lack of vegetation or very high mountains, and confirmed that the dominant air currents led to an uninterrupted flow of the corrupt air from the lake into the city. After analyzing the chemical results of the water sample they took from the lake, they deduced that due to the fermentation of organic matter taking place there, the lake consumed more oxygen than the city's 350,000 inhabitants. Thus it could be construed that the lake was more harmful to the city than all the people who lived there. The results they obtained regarding the air currents confirmed that the winds took the poisonous air from the lake into the city, especially at night when the temperature decreased, and that that same air polluted aqueducts and public fountains, as well as the water consumed in homes, factories and commerce.[42]

The other adverse factor that the city faced was that its sewage system was in complete chaos. The system aimed to discharge all its refuse into Lake Texcoco. However, the floor of the city was 1.5 metres above the level of the lake, and if the water level of the lake increased, the water from the sewers could only flow back into the city.[43] Thus, the environmental threats the city faced were above all from water — tainted water. The water in the lake was full of waste, and beneath the city the land was saturated with water and criss-crossed by a deficient sewage system that was broken and/or clogged. So it is clear why the water below *la ciudad de los Palacios* — as Mexico City was called — was particularly dangerous to the health of the urban population.[44]

Not only was water a major problem, but physicians also argued that the city's atmosphere was polluted with miasmas. Thus, the persistent demands made by public health officials for the city to be cleaned, adequate sewers to be installed and excess water to be drained, as well as their demands for pure air, adequate light in all homes and clean water for the city could all be summed up in one word: hygiene.

The sixteenth-century association of Lake Texcoco with the Beast of the Apocalypse, and the fact that this lake had for centuries been seen as a source of disease, can be understood as being inscribed within the environmentalist theory of disease causation and within a mentality that found in religion and magic explanations for the cause of disease, and in particular of epidemics, since "both individual and collective sickness could be rationalized in terms of moral or religious failings."[45] However, Dr. Peñafiel's research into one of the sources of the unsanitary conditions of Mexico City corresponds to a different mentality. He no longer attributes the presence of disease to a punishment from God, to witchcraft or to immoral actions. He approaches the lake with a scientific background, for the purpose of a scientific inquiry, and identifies concrete elements within the lake that he believes are at the heart of the lack of an adequate level of health befitting a civilized city, and describes them. However, the fact that he resorts to emphasizing the detrimental effect of the atmosphere, and to underlining the importance of air currents and pure water for the health of the city, highlights a number of emphases: the continuing predominance of environmental explanations in the struggle to understand the causes of disease; the association between dirt and disease; and the importance that cleanliness had acquired for a city that aimed to avoid the spread of disease.

Thus, Peñafiel's expedition, as well as the opinions expressed by other public health officials, point to the fact that the "definitive secularization"[46] of the concept of infection following the discovery of bacteria as a specific etiological agent had still not permeated the cultural world of Mexican physicians of the final decades of the nineteenth century. According to Alain Corbin, before the triumph of Louis Pasteur's theories during the 1890s, doctors exercised — not without errors — an olfactory vigilance, which at times was translated into scientific language. The aim of this vigilance was varied: "to detect irrespirable gases and particularly 'airs', and to discern and describe hitherto imperceptible viruses, miasmas, and poisons."[47] However, some hygienists also began to use in their writings and explanations a discourse that emerged from the scientific breakthroughs made during the period, and Raigosa clearly exemplifies this trend. For him, the admirable scientific discoveries recently made by Louis Pasteur in France had led to the opening of an infinite horizon, "to the penetrant gaze of the microscope, which has made visible a world of organisms that pervade the air, the water and the land."[48] Raigosa stressed that it was well known that two types of microscopic organisms existed, those that caused no harm to man or to any living animal or plant, and those that caused disease to all living things. The deadly microscopic organisms were included in the category of decay, putrefaction and fermentation, and hygienists devised a new category of diseases, the so-called 'zymotic' diseases.[49] This term reflected the idea of the disease process as being analogous to fermentation, and included cholera, typhoid, diphtheria, smallpox, measles and scarlet fever.[50] These diseases — some hygienists and physicians believed — were introduced into the human body by drinking tainted water or by inhaling the miasmatic emanations that emerged from sites of decomposition and fermentation, such as marshes and stagnant water.[51] Thus, by the 1880s, the predominant explanation of disease causation still held miasmas responsible, regardless of the fact that the existence of microorganisms was known.

The acceptance of the germ theory of disease — a watershed in medical history — was neither immediate nor general among the scientific community of the time. Its acceptance was gradual, and contemporaries considered it one of many theories that had to be debated and proved. [52] For instance, in 1885, two years after the German physician Robert Koch identified the pathogenic organism of cholera, Dr. Manuel de la Fuente held that the discoveries made by Koch were not unquestionable truths for science.[53] The same view was expressed in 1884 and 1889 by the Superior Sanitation Council, when it asserted that the unsanitary conditions of Mexico City had their origin in miasmas.[54]

Of particular importance for this study is the fact that the germ theory of disease reinforced to a large degree the assumptions of the environmental theories of disease causation by confirming the risks of polluted water, lack of personal hygiene and overcrowded conditions. Thus, before the widespread acceptance of the germ theory of disease, the experts continued to stress the need to ameliorate the environment. This is precisely what was taking place in Mexico City, and the figures that showed the rate of premature death in the city made it vitally important to improve the environment.

According to the statistical information presented by Raigosa, between 1867 and 1877, a total of 83,043 people had died of preventable diseases in the city, which at that time had a population of approximately 250,000.[55] This meant that one third of the capital's population had been lost in only a decade, and if it had not been for the rural-urban migration the city would have had hardly any inhabitants left. In 1876, one out of every nineteen people died prematurely in the city. When this figure was compared to the statistical information available on other parts of the world, it only served to confirm the grim conditions that prevailed. Raigosa noted that in England, one out of every fifty-two inhabitants died prematurely; in France one out of every forty-four, in Spain one out of every thirty-four. This provided numerical evidence that the capital city of Mexico was the most unsanitary region in the world.

Ensuring the people's health was not merely necessary for their own well-being; it was also important in terms of economic development and national defence. Public health had become a national quest, one that in the particular case of Mexico equated nation with capital city. Thus, physicians, state agencies and sanitary engineers argued that it was absolutely imperative to make the city a healthy place to live, and that the only way that this could be done was by expelling all visible water and by draining the water below the surface. The mission of sanitary engineers and hygienists can be summed up in the following words:

> To sanitize this lethal city! ...To restore to the atmosphere its purity; to the land its fecundity, to the climate its mildness, to the vegetation its splendor, to the race its lost vitality, to human life its normal development.[56]

Elements of a Healthy City

If the environment was harmful to the population, what characteristics should a healthy city have? Dr. Luis E. Ruiz, in his *Tratado elemental de higiene* (1904), detailed all the necessary requirements if a city was to control the threats posed by its environment. Ruiz (1857–1914) was one of the most prestigious and influential doctors during the Díaz regime and was also an advocate of scientific politics. Between 1878 and 1884, he was the scientific editor of *La Libertad,* the newspaper that presented the notion of scientific politics as a new and regenerating doctrine in Mexico. He was a member of the *Asociación Metodófila Gabino Barreda*, a short-lived association formed by twenty-five students — mostly of medicine — whose task was to apply the rigorous logic of the scientific method to every kind of phenomenon. He also participated at the Second Congress of Public Instruction (29 November 1890 to 28 February 1891), and in 1896 was director of the General Board of Primary Education (Dirección General de Instrucción Primaria).[57] Ruiz wrote extensively about typhus, vaccination (smallpox and rabies), the benefits of a healthy diet, and about the importance of water for a healthy constitution, and authored the books *Tratado elemental de pedagogía* (1900), and *Guía de la ciudad de México* (1910), among others. He worked in the Hospital Juárez, was a member of the National Academy of Medicine and its director as of 1898, and was one of the most respected members of the Superior Sanitation Council.[58] In the *Tratado elemental de Higiene*, he categorically affirmed that hygiene was the scientific art of preserving health and increasing prosperity, and that all civilized nations had as their principal interest public health. According to Ruiz, all administrative and economic policies were inseparable from hygienic issues.[59]

Ruiz believed that life in a city was the best possible life, and that the city was the collective home of the human race. The city was, in addition, the physical and moral site where men could best develop, progress and become good and healthy citizens.[60] However, all cities had to fulfill a number of conditions in order to overcome the damaging effects that any numerous congregation of individuals were bound to have upon life in an urban space. Any mass of people would foul the land, alter the air and pollute the water. Therefore, the adequate cleansing of the city was the axis of urban hygiene, argued Ruiz, quoting Dr. Fonssagrives, one of the most influential French hygienists of the nineteenth century.

The first step in improving urban hygiene in Mexico City was to make sure that the excess water was efficiently drained from the subsoil, that all human waste was taken away from populated areas and that waterproof paving was laid on as many streets as possible. However, the most efficient way of dealing with both excess water and human waste — the former being the result of the unfortunate location of the city and the latter a consequence of both the natural environment and urban growth — was by building a proper drainage system.[61] The construction of a drainage system for the city would make it a safe and comfortable place, and everything detrimental to the senses and to health would be effectively removed. The drainage or disappearance of all the excess water from beneath the city, water that was both impure and foul-smelling, not only would benefit public health, but would also facilitate the physical expansion of the city. If the land was dry, buildings could be constructed without fear for their structures; roads could be extended; rail tracks could have a safer foundation. The construction of a drainage system was thus seen as a material factor, the fruition of science and engineering that would improve the urban infrastructure and the quality of life.

Another key factor in developing a clean city was the availability of numerous green areas, parks and gardens that would not only enhance the visual environment but also contribute to the health of the population. In 1892, Dr. Jesús Alfaro's thesis for the National School of Medicine, entitled *Higiene pública: Algunas palabras acerca de la influencia higiénica de las arboledas y necesidad de reglamentar su uso entre nosotros*, advised that the city should have as many green areas as possible, not only because they were required for beauty and embellishment, but also because they were indeed crucial to hygiene.[62] He believed that trees would absorb the underground water from the city's subsoil and help to transform marshes into gardens. It was a scientific fact, he argued, that trees purified the air, ridding the atmosphere of miasmas, that they kept an atmospheric balance that would prevent sudden changes in temperature, and defined them as "instruments of disinfection."[63] He urged the government to create a special commission exclusively devoted to assessing the hygienic benefits of green areas for the city and criticized the unrestrained destruction of the city's vegetation as a result of the "construction of railways," one of the most cherished symbols of progress.[64]

Engineer Miguel Angel de Quevedo was also a keen advocate of the benefits of green areas for the hygiene and beauty of a city. Quevedo had studied engineering in Paris, attended numerous international conferences on urban hygiene and city planning, and the model of urban planning he favoured for Mexico City was the Parisian example. Its long diagonal avenues, its *rond points* and numerous green areas, if applied to Mexico, would transform "our beloved capital" into the "Paris of America." He imagined a comprehensive urban park system aimed at creating gardens and parks throughout the city, some of which would be built exclusively for the urban working class, such as the Balbuena Park (inaugurated in 1910). Quevedo held that Mexico City ranked last among "selected capitals of the world in terms of inhabitants per park acre — 1 hectare for 2500 residents, as compared to Washington, DC, which provided 1 hectare for 206 residents." The benefits accruing to the city from numerous green areas linked hygiene with beauty, and according to Quevedo, Mexico City was responsible for the "pallid color and more or less sickly and anemic state of the capital's inhabitants."[65]

Another basic necessity for a city in control of its environment was the availability of abundant drinking water. Water was important to all the inhabitants because most social, commercial, industrial and hygienic activities required it; and it could also be used to channel all the refuse and human waste in the drains out of the city.[66] Impure water must be prevented from assaulting the senses of the city's inhabitants, and pure water had to be made available to the entire city via adequate water conduits established in all homes. Aqueducts, wells, public fountains and water-carriers were all ways of supplying water which were incompatible with health; drinking water had to be introduced to all homes via enclosed and invisible underground conduits. The city also had to have public bathrooms, as well as public wash-houses, efficient systems of waste collection and disposal and a guaranteed abundant food supply.[67]

Ruiz believed that cleanliness was the most important element in developing a hygienic and ordered city, and made the following distinction: personal cleanliness was the duty of the individual, the cleanliness of the home was the responsibility of the family, and the cleanliness of the city was the responsibility of the communal authority.[68] For Eduardo Liceaga, all that was required to avoid becoming a victim of disease could be summed up in a single word: cleanliness. In 1895, another physician, Domingo Orvañanos, stated that cleanliness was the most important element for a healthy constitution and for a healthy city.[69] The association of cleanliness with health, both private and public, is the most persistent assumption in the discourse about the city during the final decades of the nineteenth century. Cleanliness was associated with health and order; dirt was associated with disorder. Mary Douglas has analyzed in great detail the different dialectics of the pure and the impure, as well as the logic behind the dangers of defilement. When apparent disorder reigns in a given society — she has stated — dirt is identified as a matter out of place, as a threat to order, and is "vigorously brushed away."[70] The creation of frontiers, barriers and exclusions when referring to the clean/unclean can be clearly appreciated in the following statement made by Domingo Orvañanos. His perception of the dangers posed to Mexican society relies on identifying a specific component of the Mexican population as an imminent threat: "Mortality is higher where the indigenous race predominates. This is due to their lack of cleanliness."[71]

Thus, the indigenous population of Mexico was associated with uncleanness and rejected. The threat to the health of the city was therefore latent not only in the environment, but also in every house, and the home became one of the places targeted by the recommendations of hygienists. Their goal was to free all homes of dirt, because each and every house was a possible focus of disease.[72] Houses — inside and out — had to be clean, free of litter and waste, and provided with sufficient and pure water. In addition, the cleansing of the body had to be practised with care and dedication, everyone had to try to have a bath in cold water every day and have a healthy diet, all activities, whether to do with work, leisure or sex, had to be moderate, and all excesses had to be avoided.[73]

The emphasis placed on personal and household hygiene was inexorably linked to the gradual acceptance of the germ theory of disease. As the theory gained adherents within the medical establishment, articles about the germ theory began to reach Mexico City's limited reading public via newspapers and magazines.[74] The authors of those articles — newspaper reporters, physicians, hygienists, women and writers — informed the men, women and children of the numerous invisible threats to health present in all households and bodies, but the old idea that miasmas caused disease lingered, and on many occasions the concepts of germs and miasmas were used interchangeably.[75]

Mexico City embodied during the final decades of the nineteenth century an unresolved contradiction. The capital of the country, the centre of culture, civilization, economic and political power, was corrupted, dirty, foul-smelling and dangerous, and this was evident not only among the urban population but within the environment itself. What physicians, hygienists and sanitary engineers wanted was to attain a "vision of a society renovated by renovation of the urban infrastructure below ground and above."[76] Thus, physicians and engineers created a discourse about the city in which hygiene, health, morality, order and cleanliness were woven together as goals to be achieved, and the threat posed to the city (civilization) by the proximity of an untamed environment and by its inhabitants (barbarism) had to be dealt with. Through the use of statistical information, public health officials analyzed everything that might lead to illness or premature death. These diagnoses contrasted with the pleasures that Macedo believed were present in the capital and which, according to him, attracted so many people from other parts of the country.

3

The Expansion and Diagnosis of the City

The Expansion of the City

In October 1884, the Mexico City's Municipal Council acknowledged that it was absolutely necessary to have an up-to-date map of the city, and argued that even though the 1871 map had been appropriate in its time, "today it is incomplete due to the changes the city experienced in the past thirteen years; the construction of new streets, neighborhoods and buildings have transformed its features and physiognomy."[1] The physical expansion of the city, the creation of a communications infrastructure and the construction of new residential areas, or *colonias*, altered the capital in a radical way during the Porfiriato. This expansion was closely linked to the integration of Mexico into the world economy after 1870, during the phase of export-led growth (between 1870 and the World Depression of 1929–33), a development that had profound effects upon most Latin American capital cities.[2] According to María Dolores Morales, Mexico City was subject to three phases of growth, two of them during the second half of the nineteenth century (1858–83 and 1884–89) and the third during the first decade of the twentieth century (1900–10). In 1858, the city occupied an area of 8.5 square kilometres; by 1910, it covered 40.5 square kilometres, while the urban population more than doubled between 1858 and 1910: from two hundred thousand inhabitants to 471,066 in 1910.[3] And it was precisely during those years that thirty-four residential areas were built, most of them after 1884 and in particular during the first decade of the twentieth century (see Table 1).

Table 1: Expansion of Mexico City, 1858–1910

First phase, 1858–83	Second phase, 1884–89	Third phase, 1900–10
1. Barroso	1. Morelos	1. La Teja
2. Sta. María	2. La Bolsa	1.1 Americana
3. Arquitectos	3. Díaz de León	1.2 Juárez
4. Guerrero	4. Maza	1.3 Cuauhtémoc
5. Violante	5. Rastro	2. Roma
	6. Valle Gómez	3. Condesa
	7. San Rafael	4. Tlaxpana
	8. Sta. Julia	5. Sto. Tomás
	9. Limantour	6. Chopo
	10. Indianilla	7. San Alvaro
	11. Hidalgo	8. El Imparcial
	12. Ampliación Sta. María (Ladrillera)	9. Peralvillo
		10. Cuartelito
		11. La Viga
		12. Scheibe
		13. Romero Rubio
		14. Ampliación San Rafael (La Blanca)

Source: María Dolores Morales, "La expansión de la ciudad de México (1858–1910)," in *Atlas de la Ciudad de México*, edited by Gustavo Garza (Mexico City: Departamento del Distrito Federal – El Colegio de México, 1987), 67.

The symbolic significance of this expansion, that is, the incorporation or colonization of previously excluded rural areas into the fabric of the city, can be found in the name given to them — *colonias* — and in the fact that the aim was to transform the agricultural regions — the countryside — so that they ceased to be "empty" and "backward." This incorporation of previously excluded areas reflects the way in which the physical borders of the city were being redefined or redrawn. The request made by the Municipal Council in 1884 for an adequate map of the city clearly points to the fact that the limits of the city were changing. This process of frontier expansion took place at a time when economic and political power was becoming increasingly centralized in Mexico City, when the city was associated with political peace and social order, and when issues relating to health were acquiring a particular prominence.

The expansion of the city took place as the Porfirian regime secured the political and economic domination of the city over the rest of the nation and the capital became the privileged site where the modernity of the nation had to be visible, tangible and on display. The city had to be seen as the modern capital of a country that — it was said — was steadily achieving progress, and thus the thrust of public health measures involved improving hygiene and sanitation. This implied that the city and its inhabitants had to be clean, ordered and hygienic; epidemic and non-epidemic diseases had to be controlled, and health-enhancing elements such as green areas, adequately paved streets and efficient sewers, among others, had to be introduced. This concern with public health and sanitation was also a major issue in other Latin American cities during the final decades of the nineteenth century, when it became crucial to modernize the capital cities by eradicating sources of disease in order to increase the labour supply and attract foreign immigrants and capital. The eradication of sources of disease became a crucial element in the discourse on the modern city, and in the policies that aimed to transform its sanitary conditions, its functioning and its appearance.[4] It should be stressed that the beginnings of modern health policy in Latin American cities often coincided with the genesis of modern policing and detection methods, each being seen as means by which society could be sanitized in the name of progress.[5] The city's progress, according to the Porfirian elite, meant that its modernity had to be on display, and all that impinged negatively upon public health eradicated. However, the expansion of the city was neither uniform nor thoroughly planned, and it certainly did not mean that once the space was incorporated into the urban domain, its physiognomy ceased to be rural and acquired a distinctive "urban" or "modern" character. It should be remembered that the country in 1910 was predominantly rural, and that even within the city the rural milieu persisted. This meant that new and old cultural influences continuously collided in the streets of the capital and that in spite of the creation of the *colonias*, large areas within the city continued to be used for agriculture and for raising cattle. Many of the migrants who arrived in the city throughout the Díaz regime brought with them their material belongings, but also their customs, traditions and beliefs, as well as their social practices; the city was both urban and rural.

When positive comments were made about the city, what was praised as modern and comfortable was a very small proportion of its area, namely the better urbanized *colonias* and specific roads or avenues that were embellished by the erection of statues, parks and historical monuments, where the well-to-do sectors of the urban population could stroll on any Sunday afternoon without having their *paseo* ruined by the presence of badly dressed and foul-smelling people. However, the city also possessed a number of features that were considered absolutely incompatible with the image of modernity the Porfirian elite was so eager to promote: the presence of tainted water, the dirtiness of the streets, the poor hygienic practices of many of the inhabitants, and the threats posed both to the image of modernity and to public health by its unsanitary conditions.

During the first phase of frontier expansion (1858–83), the city's growth was slow. There was neither a considerable natural population growth nor substantial immigration. Many of the city's inhabitants lived in the central district, and the expansion was largely the result of the impact of the Leyes de Desamortización or Ley Lerdo (1856) and of the Laws of Reform (12 July 1859). These laws led to the incorporation and commercialization of land and property that had belonged to the Catholic Church, such as schools, convents and cemeteries, and to the commercialization of communal land belonging to the indigenous population. The latter, as Andrés Lira has shown, caused the destruction of communities and livelihoods.[6] Another factor that contributed to this initial phase of physical expansion was the drainage of canals, swamps and marshes surrounding the urban area, which made possible the establishment of a communications infrastructure, in particular the construction of railways and rail tracks.[7] But the direction of expansion of the city was also determined by the quality of the land. The areas to the east, in particular those closer to Lake Texcoco, became the least favoured sites for the construction of housing areas. The continuous threat of overflow from the lake, as well as the stench that emanated from the city's cesspool, simply did not encourage investors.

The five *colonias* created between 1858 and 1883 occupied areas to the northeast of the Plaza Mayor or Zócalo (Barroso, Santa María and Guerrero); to the west (*colonia* Arquitectos) and to the northwest (*colonia* Violante), and were built with a clear intention as to which sectors of the urban population should inhabit them. This represented a radical rupture with the way in which the city had been inhabited or occupied since the seventeenth century, when the urban population had not been segregated along socio-economic lines.[8] The *colonia* Santa María was built to house sectors of the urban middle class, in particular lawyers and merchants; the *colonia* Guerrero was created for the urban working class, and the *colonia* Arquitectos was planned to house the architects of the city.[9] This deliberate segregation of the urban population became more pronounced during the second phase of expansion, and in particular during the first decade of the twentieth century, and led to the creation of two cities within the capital. One was the "modern" city, inhabited by a minority of the urban population and located to the southeast of the Plaza Mayor; the other was the chaotic city, which remained at the margins of the modern capital. This marginal city became the focus of attention for sanitary inspectors in their attempt to transform not only the physical environment but also its dwellers.

Between 1884 and 1899, twelve *colonias* were created, with the largest urban developments appearing in the northeast, where the *colonias* Morelos, La Bolsa, Díaz de León, Rastro, Maza and Valle Gómez were built. These housing areas were for urban workers with scarce resources, and their creation was propelled by the construction in this same area of the Penitenciaría (city jail),[10] the city's slaughterhouse (Rastro), the Estación de Hidalgo and the railway tracks of the Ferrocarriles Guadalupe, Interoceánico and Cintura, where the inhabitants of these *colonias* often worked.[11] To the east, sectors of the urban middle class settled in the *colonia* San Rafael, and the *colonia* Santa Julia — also to the east — was referred to as a "colonia popular." To the south, the *colonias* Limantour, Indianilla and Hidalgo appeared. The indigenous communities remained neglected at the edges of the city, in *barrios*, not in *colonias*.

The seventeen incorporated or colonized regions that emerged between 1858 and 1899 were often built by individuals with limited resources who invested in real estate or built houses and communication infrastructures. In addition, the Municipal Council, attempting to address the city's lack of resources, gave individuals ample freedom and numerous facilities to help in incorporating new areas into the city. These individuals benefited from generous tax exemptions, and had access to building materials free of tax. However, because there were no clear policies or guidelines to follow, and because the provision of public services was not a requirement either of the promoters or the Municipal Council, the new urban developments were not afforded services such as sewers, drainage, paved streets and drinking water.

Land speculation also became an increasingly profitable business. Due to changes in the use of land, now used to promote housing areas, industries, commerce and/or communication infrastructure, the price of land increased. For instance, the cost of plots of land on the Paseo de la Reforma in 1872 was 1.50 pesos per square metre, and by 1903 the cost had risen to twenty-five pesos per square metre. Land in the *colonia* Santa María was initially sold at 0.27 pesos per square metre, and by 1901 at fifteen pesos. In 1872, two years before the *colonia* Guerrero was created, the price of an agricultural plot of land was 0.02 pesos per square metre; by 1901 (as a housing area), the price had increased to 13.04 pesos per square metre. The value of land in the centre of the city also increased dramatically, and this made peripheral areas more attractive for the promoters of new residential areas. In 1901, land in the central streets of the city cost between eighty and 160 pesos per square metre, and the price of land in new housing areas during that same year, in the suburbs and with no public services, ranged between 2.50 and twenty pesos per square metre.[12]

The incorporation of new areas into the city was determined by the cost and quality of the land, by the proximity these new *colonias* would have to transport facilities, such as roads, railway stations and rail tracks, and by their distance from Lake Texcoco. The west and southwest became the privileged sites for urban expansion, and the east remained a marginal area. Poorer sectors of the urban population lived in the east and northeast, areas that were permanently threatened by the overflow of Lake Texcoco. By contrast, to the west and southwest, where the land was drier and less prone to the impact of periodic floods, sectors of the urban population could live without fear of the invasion of tainted water. The southwest became the favoured site where the Porfirian elite gradually settled, abandoning the traditional locus of power, the area surrounding the Plaza Mayor.

What distinguished the first two phases of expansion from the years between 1900 and 1910 was that during the first decade of the twentieth century, the expansion was driven not by private individuals with little capital, but by private companies supported by banks.[13] This led to the creation of some housing areas destined exclusively for the well-to-do sectors of the urban population, such as the *colonias* Juárez, Cuauhtémoc, Roma and Condesa in the southwest. Additionally, in 1903, the Municipal Council set down a number of requirements that had to be followed when creating new housing areas. For instance, it specified the width and length all streets should have, the number of blocks each new housing area must posses, and that a garden or plaza had to be present. In addition, drinking water availability and sewers had to be thoroughly planned.[14]

Mexico City, like other Latin American cities of the period, experienced selective and pragmatic urban changes that were partly inspired by the changes carried out in Paris under the leadership of George Eugène Haussmann[15] and in the United States and Britain through the building of "garden cities." The emphasis on creating wide and long streets and avenues to ease the circulation of people and vehicles, as well as the creation of gardens, plazas and efficient public services, were all crucial elements for the modern city, not only in Mexico, but also in Rio de Janeiro and Buenos Aires.[16] However, because the urban population was swelling, other housing areas were required for the urban working class, such as the *colonia* Scheibe in the east and the *colonia* Peralvillo in the northeast.[17]

As has already been mentioned, a factor that contributed to the expansion of the city during this phase of export-led growth was the construction of a communications infrastructure, and the point of departure of all the railways was the capital of the country. Their construction stimulated the creation of housing areas and factories on the periphery of the city and allowed for additional mobility for the urban and rural population, for foodstuffs and for industrial and mineral products.[18] The visual impact of the new communications structures on the expanding city led some observers to define the changes with optimism and awe:

> It is just nightfall, one of the times when most movement can be observed in the streets: thousands of workers have just left work and the streets are swarming with people, whether one looks toward the outskirts or toward the downtown avenues. The entire city is crisscrossed by rails, on which the street cars run, leading to the modern *colonias* or to more distant sites, or to neighbouring *pueblos*; passenger cars move along incessantly, most of them pulled by starving, old hacks; the elegant carriages belonging to distinguished or well-to-do families return from

the Bosque de Chapultepec and from the Paseo de la Reforma; the commercial houses of Plateros, Refugio, Cinco de Mayo and adjacent streets are lavishly illuminated; thousands of confused murmurs, thousands of mutters float in the air, the clamour of the populace, the noise of the vehicles, the whistle of the trains, the resounding bugle of the barracks, these are just some of the many echoes of the busy life of large cities.[19]

The previous passage portrays the city as full of life, noise, movement and people, with numerous rail tracks and vehicles criss-crossing it. However, it also indicates the segregation of the urban population. Some people are described as leaving their work and going to the most distant sites (they could be the *colonias* La Bolsa and Rastro), while others made their way to the modern *colonias* (definitively Juárez and Cuauhtémoc). Where you lived and how you lived in Mexico City increasingly became, during the course of the second half of the nineteenth century, an expression of the social and cultural milieu to which you belonged.[20]

This segregation of the urban population meant that the best and most modern *colonias*, that is, those inhabited by the richest sectors of the urban population, gradually acquired most public services, such as paved streets, transport, water and sewers. However, most areas of the city remained excluded from the elements the Porfirian elite described or made reference to as the material evidence of the modernity of the capital. The expansion of the city led not only to the creation of spatial frontiers within it, but also to the perception of the capital as being made up of different and exclusive entities. Thus, the city of the Porfirio Díaz regime was characterized by the creation of both material and discursive boundaries and exclusions. In 1908, for example, the city was described as follows:

> Mexico is made up of three parts: an *ancient Mexico*, the Mexico of our grandparents, purely colonial, with its ancestral homes, its large tenement buildings, its slums, its legends, traditions, its old-fashioned flavor and unquestionable delights; a completely new Mexico, built in-between; and a *modern Mexico*, incrusted in the first, with its *barrios* transformed as a result of the sanitation works, its large and luxurious department stores and the clamor of contemporary life, pure commotion, nerves, fast and bustling.[21]

The creation of physical, material and discursive frontiers reinforced the cultural and social and economic segregation of the urban population. This erection of frontiers reinforced the elites' perception that it was vital to assimilate and incorporate the backward areas surrounding the modern city through their absorption into the fabric of civilized society. And one of the elements that would allow their incorporation was hygiene. "Ancient" Mexico was habitually defined as dirty, health-endangering, foul-smelling and vice-ridden, and was seen as a threat to the civilizing endeavours of public health officials, while the eastern area became the prototype of ancient Mexico and the southwest the prototype of modern Mexico. [22]

Throughout the course of the nineteenth century, numerous laws were passed specifying the measures that had to be implemented to keep the city clean, many of which had been established since the late colonial period. In 1834, for example, José María Tornel published a *bando de policía* in which he made reference to the laws of 1780, 1790, 1791, 1796, and particularly to one issued in 1822. All of these laws embraced most of the issues that had to be considered in cleansing the city and improving its sanitary conditions. The intention of the 1822 law was much the same as what was attempted during the Porfiriato: all streets, public fountains and public areas should be adequately cleansed, all street vendors should clean the streets after selling their products; all the inhabitants of the city had to clean the front of their houses and collect all rubbish and fecal waste from the gutters and open ditches.[23] During the final decades of the nineteenth century, it was argued that in spite of legislation that prohibited the creation of waste dumps in areas not designated for this purpose, and that made clear that no fecal waste or dead animals should be dumped in them, waste was generally disposed of in any place found convenient by the *citadinos*. Therefore, it was not unusual for foreigners to see the city, including the central area, looking like a disgusting waste site.[24] In 1886, a *Bando sobre aseo de las vías públicas de la ciudad de México* was published, and its fourteen sections detailed the provisions all city dwellers had to comply with in an effort to keep the city clean, tidy and hygienic, establishing in addition fines and penalties for anyone found to be urinating in public areas.[25] The regulations were to be followed throughout the city, but the eastern sector was of particular concern, not only because it lacked the most basic public services, but also because of its proximity to Lake Texcoco.

As has been shown, the expansion of the city was primarily towards the west, north and south, not towards the east. The eastern area of the city was at a lower altitude than the rest of the city, its land was rich in saltpetre, and it was too close to Lake Texcoco. It was well known that whenever it rained heavily, all areas close to the cesspool of the city were bound to become fully submerged in it. The eastern area of the city remained neglected and did not become a place of interest, either for basic urban infrastructure or for the creation of comfortable houses. In addition, it was inhabited primarily by poor sectors of the urban population.[26]

The presence of tainted water inside the city, on its streets, canals and aqueducts, was a problem that had to be addressed. Even though many of the canals that crossed the city had been drained and covered during the eighteenth and nineteenth centuries, some still remained during the Porfiriato. Canals and aqueducts were seen as dangerous to public health. Many people used the canals to dispose of all their litter and waste, and it was argued that they fouled both water and air. Aqueducts were said to carry tainted water, and were regarded not only as health-endangering elements, but also as a physical obstacle to the expansion of the city and to the construction of roads, avenues and rail tracks. Nature was seen as an element that had to be dominated, controlled and civilized. The expansion of the city meant civilization, inclusion and order, and the canals that swept along litter and disease, as well as the people who used them as a means of transport to travel from the outskirts into the central markets to sell their fruit, vegetables and flowers, had to go.

The desire to tame, civilize or incorporate nature was ultimately linked to the idea of creating a hygienic city, and was not exclusive to Mexico City. In Buenos Aires, the construction of a hygienic city began in 1874, after the devastating impact of a yellow fever epidemic that swept across the city in 1871. In July 1871, five months after the epidemic, Domingo F. Sarmiento said it was crucial to expel all water from the city, and believed that the construction of efficient public services would make the city a healthy environment.[27] In Mexico City, it was said that the "mud and stagnant water mired the dictatorship's silver dollar wheels,"[28] and in 1878, the press compared Mexico City to the sea: "the city is a port without a beach."[29] In October 1886, most of the city became a huge lake when more than five hundred homes were flooded and eight collapsed, many central streets became putrid lakes that interrupted traffic and gave off a terrible stench causing nausea among the city's inhabitants.[30] Due to the chaos caused by the floods, a new occupation arose in Mexico City: that of people who carried others across the streets and charged fifty cents for this service. When water reclaimed the city, it blurred those precise and distinct margins between the city and the countryside that the Porfirian elite wanted to see in place, making nature a threat to the inhabitants and the built environment.[31]

The city's odours had an important significance, and some had to be eradicated. In the book *El Cuarto Poder*, written in 1888 by the journalist, politician and writer Emilio Rabasa, the first chapter is named "La Ciudad de los Palacios," and the following is the story narrated in its opening paragraphs. Juan de Quiñones is resting in his room trying to get some sleep, and the sound of an imminent storm makes him remember and feel nostalgia for his life in the countryside. But suddenly he is brought back to reality, to Mexico City and he asks himself: "Where is this stench coming from? Good bye countryside, flowers, clouds and scented earth. A terrible stench, capable of producing nausea and something even more serious suddenly brought me back to the grotesque reality that surrounded me."[32] Juan de Quiñones goes to the room next to his and asks Don Ambrosio why there is such a stench:

> But tell me, why is there this stench throughout the house?
>
> Well, because it rains — answered Don Ambrosio.
>
> Because it rains? — he replied in disbelief.
>
> Its the sewers — the old man replied — the street sewers. The fact is that the city has no drainage system, and neither does the Valley of Mexico, and it shall possess none until the mob that calls itself Liberal ceases to govern the country. Mexico is the most important city of Latin America ... Foreigners become truly admired when they come to the city. And if when it rains there is a bad smell, it is not the city's fault but the fault of those that do not cleanse it.[33]

The earlier explanation of how when it rained all the images of the modern city suddenly collapsed in the face of a terrible smell that permeated everything reflects a real problem: the stench that invaded the city whenever the rain was heavy enough to make its sewers overflow. This sensitivity to odours was shared by many doctors who inspected the city and Lake Texcoco, and bad odours had for a very long time been thought to be a cause of disease. Thus, the aim of creating an odourless city was linked to the need to prevent disease and ultimately premature death, but it also represented a sort of revolution in civic cleanliness which entailed radical changes in personal cleanliness. So, just as some visual elements within the urban space had to go or change, odours which disturbed and caused headaches, nausea or illness had to be suppressed.

Doctors and hygienists had to make sure that the urban population did what was recommended by the dictates of hygiene. This implied a more thorough control of the activities, social practices and customs of the urban population. The cleansing of the city, the creation of boundaries between what was permissible and what was not, had an impact on urban planning and design: the thrust was to create a city wherein each activity had a specific place designated for that specific purpose. All of this took place — as we have seen — at a time when the city was expanding physically and the population was increasing. Thus, in order to control many of the unsanitary features of the city and to find a definitive solution, a thorough investigation of the Capital was required. To this end, the role played by the members of the Superior Sanitation Council was paramount.

Public health officials — as has been mentioned — emerged from different disciplines, and they managed to create a discourse about the city and its inhabitants in which the notions of order, cleanliness and hygiene were regarded as indispensable for a comfortable, safe and modern city. Their recommendations embraced both health issues and the need to educate the urban population; thus public health encompassed a moral and an educational dimension.[34] Public health officials (hygienists, physicians, engineers, architects and state agencies), and in particular the members of the Superior Sanitation Council, contributed their expertise and prestige to a project which aimed to create a truly modern city, and to this end they instigated broad socio-medical investigations of the city and its inhabitants.

The Superior Sanitation Council and the Sanitary Code

The Superior Sanitation Council was the body responsible for all public health and sanitation issues, and the city became the focus of investigation of the numerous commissions that formed it. It was made up not only of doctors or hygienists, but also included architects and engineers, and the Ministry of the Interior and the Municipal Council were actively involved. Engineers and architects embarked on the construction of railroads, ports, canals, mines, industries, monuments and infrastructural works, such as the drainage system. It was believed that the drainage system would protect the capital from flooding and contribute to its transformation into a clean and hygienic city.[35] However, along with the construction of this major public work, it was imperative to control the unsanitary conditions in the city by forcing its inhabitants to comply with the precepts that hygiene dictated.[36]

Physicians and engineers were among the most prestigious professionals who had a keen interest in transforming these unsanitary conditions. Engineering was one of the most favoured professions,[37] and physicians were also highly praised, although their number was very small: out of a national population of 13,607,257 Mexicans in 1900, only 2,626 belonged to the medical profession.[38] Most worked in the capital city, but not all belonged to the Superior Sanitation Council.

One of the responsibilities of the members of the SSC was to draw up detailed maps or diagnostics of the city and to ensure that their recommendations were effectively and efficiently followed. These studies described all the sanitary problems they encountered during their inspections, and through them it is possible to visualize the model of the ideal city they aimed at attaining in conjunction with the work done by engineers, architects and state agencies. However, before discussing the information they produced, it is important to briefly sketch how the Council was organized and what activities it was involved in.

The Superior Sanitation Council was created on 4 January 1841 to replace the Medical Faculty of the Federal District. It consisted of three doctors, one pharmacist and one chemist, and its president was the governor of the Department of Mexico. Its activities included making sure that practising doctors were adequately qualified; indicating what activities phlebotomists, dentists and midwives could be engaged in; and supervising the quality of medicines produced and sold. It also had to have a close working relationship with the Municipal Council, visit hospitals, jails and schools and assess their sanitary conditions and functions. The members of the Superior Sanitation Council proposed that each district of the city should have a practising doctor whose duties would include providing medical care during normal times and during epidemics and surveying the sanitary conditions of all districts of the city. An important factor in facilitating those objectives was the division of the city into administrative and fiscal spatially circumscribed units — *cuarteles* — in 1782. During the late nineteenth century, this division continued, and it was precisely through this geographical partitioning that the members of the Superior Sanitation Council intended to detect all that was or could be a threat to public health.[39]

What began in 1841 was a deliberate attempt to supervise all matters that could impinge negatively on public health. The drawing up of medical topographies of each of the eight major quarters of the city required thorough observations concerning "the region, housing, people, principal interests, dress, atmospheric constitution [as well as the] physical and moral education of the inhabitants in [a given] area."[40] Under the constant medical scrutiny of the various activities and characteristics of urban life, the writing and diffusion of codes became fundamental and was linked to the collective life of the nation. Within this process, knowledge ceased to concentrate solely on curing ills, but also embraced the study of the healthy man, that is, the non-sick man, and led to a definition of the model man.[41]

In Mexico, the writing and diffusion of codes implied the intervening power of a medical gaze upon society, and this can be seen in the 1872 decree issued by the Ministry of the Interior establishing the *Reglamento del Consejo Superior de Salubridad*. These regulations asserted that among its multiple tasks the SSC was responsible for creating medical statistics, and that, using the data gathered and the detailed observations of the city, it had to propose specific measures for public and private hygiene.[42]

During the first presidency of General Porfirio Díaz (23 November 1876 to 30 November 1880), the Superior Sanitation Council briefly ceased to be part of the Ministry of the Interior and was placed under the Junta Directiva de Beneficencia (from 23 January 1877 to 1 July 1879). However, a decree was issued on 30 June 1879 which stated that the Superior Sanitation

Council would again be answerable to the Ministry of the Interior.[43] According to Porfirio Díaz, the respectability of the Superior Sanitation Council had been hampered when it depended on the Junta de Beneficencia, and the 1879 reform implied that the executive power, through the Ministry of the Interior, was to supervise the measures taken to remedy the unsanitary conditions of the city. The health of the city became identified as one of the major concerns of the nation.

In 1879, the Superior Sanitation Council was also reorganized, and four physicians, one pharmacist, a veterinary surgeon and six substitutes, were all directly appointed by the government. It was also subdivided into twelve permanent commissions responsible for a separate surveillance of most of the city's activities, and had eight sanitary inspectors, one for each of the eight quarters into which the city was divided. With regard to the permanent commissions, its members were responsible for sanitary conditions found in theatres, hospitals, jails and other places where people gathered; cemeteries, chemical establishments, pharmacies, and other factories and industries; stables, dairies and all aspects relative to veterinary medicine; food inspection, sanitary inspection and vaccination; as well as canals, gutters and sewers.[44] However, it must be stressed that the Superior Sanitation Council did not have jurisdiction throughout the country. Its activities were centred on the Federal District, and particularly on Mexico City. The functions and obligations of the members of the SSC went beyond informing the government of the hygienic problems faced in the city and among its inhabitants. It was allowed to act when it thought it was necessary to do so and could ask any other government department for any information it needed for its work. It also had to submit annual reports to the Ministry of the Interior, and these had to include medical statistics on the Federal District.[45]

The number of commissions of the Superior Sanitation Council rapidly multiplied in tandem with the expansion of the city. By 1900, it was subdivided into twenty-three different commissions, and the collective task they had before them was enormous.[46] This new division of the Superior Sanitation Council reflects the wide-ranging and generalized supervision that was thought desirable at the time. Through each of these commissions, it observed, classified and analyzed urban space in search of the problems that could threaten the health of the urban population and attempted to eradicate them. In addition, after

1880, the eight sanitary inspectors of the Superior Sanitation Council worked to predetermined guidelines, through a standard questionnaire that all inspectors were required to have with them during their inspections.[47] Using the information made available by the 1890 census, Table 2 shows the number of people who lived in each quarter of the city.

Each sanitary inspector made a study of the city, proposed measures to remedy and/or clean those features or areas that contributed to the spread of illness and/or premature death, and thus became an important instrument of political power. This meant that a small sector of the governing elite attempted to transform and normalize, through health measures and through the principles and precepts of personal hygiene, the urban space and its inhabitants. The control of urban space through health measures became an important component in the argument for the prosperity and order by the state and a factor that, if achieved, would make visible the material evidence of the modernity of the capital city.

The Superior Sanitation Council also published the *Boletín del Consejo Superior de Salubridad del Distrito Federal* and reported on its various activities and any scientific discovery made in any part of the world. In its first number, the editorial article introducing the journal stated that

> society, due to a universal law, the law of progress, has attempted to place the basis for a good administration ... and placing particular attention to its own preservation, has instituted scientific bodies to take care of its hygiene and of everything that relates to public health.[48]

This inevitable path of society towards progress required appropriate institutions capable of dealing with health issues — the Superior Sanitation Council — and its activities had to be supplemented by an efficient means of disseminating all relevant information. Thus, the members of the Superior Sanitation Council decided to follow the example set down by the specialized journals in Europe and the United States in an effort to make all the scientific discoveries and methods relating to public health as widely accessible as possible.[49]

Specific legislation in matters of public health and hygiene was first formulated through the Sanitary Code of the United States of Mexico (Código Sanitario de los Estados Unidos Mexicanos),

Table 2: Mexico City's population by *cuartel* according to the 1890 census

Cuartel	Population
Cuartel mayor 1	41,004
Cuartel mayor 2	66,892
Cuartel mayor 3	65,007
Cuartel mayor 4	48,155
Cuartel mayor 5	41,777
Cuartel mayor 6	34,254
Cuartel mayor 7	18,323
Cuartel mayor 8	8,953
Total	324,365

Source: "1890 Census," in *Memoria y Encuentros. La Ciudad de México y el Distrito Federal (1825–1928)*. Edited by Hira de Gortari and Regina Hernández Franyuti (Mexico City: Departamento del Distrito Federal – Instituto de Investigaciones Dr. José María Luis Mora, 1988), 281.

approved by Congress in 1891. The 1857 Constitution did not include any law relating to public health, and the Sanitary Code provided for the first time essential protection for Mexicans. It was inspired by the Sanitary Code of the State of New York, by legislation from Chile and Argentina, and by the long tradition of public health policy in France and England.[50] It was made up of four books and more than 353 articles dealing with all possible issues that could have any effect on public health. It contained specific laws that had to be followed by the Federal District and in the territories of Baja California and Tepic. It also contained precise legislation for ports and borders, but the different states of the Republic had the constitutional right and freedom to adopt these laws or to create their own sanitary codes.[51]

Mexico City had an entire book devoted to it, entitled "Sanitary Administration of the Capital of the Republic," detailing all the measures that had to be taken in the construction of homes, factories, theatres or any other place where people gathered. It also laid down standards for the commercialization of food and beverages and for hygiene in factories, industries, and all dangerous, unsanitary or uncomfortable establishments, as well as for measures that had to be taken during epidemics.[52]

The Sanitary Code clearly outlined the aims of public health officials: to create a clean, safe, hygienic city that would foster the work, enjoyment and tranquility of Mexicans and the progress of the nation. Returning to the importance of the writing and diffusion of codes that led to the institutionalization of the medical gaze, the Sanitary Code reflects this intrusive and generalized gaze on the city. Eduardo Liceaga, president of the SCC argued in 1891 that the conditions found in the city and throughout the country required that each individual sacrifice his or her own personal freedom for the benefit of the common good, and that public administration should reinforce the attainment of collective goals over individual goals.[53] To this end, and in accordance with Article 246 of the Penal Code of 1872, all public health officials who belonged to the Superior Sanitation Council had the authority to detain any individual for faults against public health and to enter any home, factory or commercial establishment while on duty.[54]

This clearly illustrates the link established at the time between public health, policing and detection, as well as the fact that it was crucial to sanitize the city.[55] The 1891 Sanitary Code established precise guidelines as to what public health officials had to search for and what measures had to be adopted, and it underwent two administrative reforms, the first in 1894 and the second in 1903.[56] Given that sanitary inspectors had the legal authority to enter any establishment or home found to be threatening, doctors acquired power. This power meant that under medical scrutiny, urban order had to coincide with the dictates of hygiene and public safety. Any individual found to be a threat to public order could be isolated from society, either by shutting off the home or building, or by placing the individual in a hospital.

In a meeting of the members of the Epidemiology Commission that took place on 22 December 1909, it was agreed that specific measures should be adopted to avoid the spreading of a typhus epidemic. Therefore, any home or room found to have someone with typhus was immediately subject to all the measures that hygiene dictated. The measures to prevent contagion were as follows: The sick had to be separated from the healthy. The room had to be cleaned, disinfected and whitened. People in contact with the sick had to be rubbed down with a substance capable of killing all parasites. The process was finished by burning all the miserable pieces of clothing and disinfecting the few articles fit to be kept rather than destroyed. If the sick person did not need to be taken to hospital, he/she had to be isolated in his/her home. The family had to maintain a general level of cleanliness inside the home, maintain adequate ventilation and comply with any suggestion or advice given by the physician responsible for that home.[57] The doctor-inspector additionally had to give the family a notice detailing the measures that had to be taken, and a notice had to be placed at the entrance of the sick-room notifying others of the possible dangers of entering.[58] Because people carrying an infectious disease were not necessarily identifiable, it was necessary to label them by placing a notice in the house or by having them confined to a restricted area. The identification of someone as a possible threat was both a preventive measure and an exclusion, a marginalization.

As can be seen from the previous pages, the work of the Superior Sanitation Council required very high standards of organization, administration and responsibility that were not always met. In addition, it required sufficient investment of capital by the government in health and sanitation. However, the allocation of resources during the final decades of the nineteenth century did not favour public health. In 1878, the government allocated 4,628 pesos to public health; by 1910, the figure had increased to 710,232. This meant that in 1878, the amount per inhabitant was 0.005 of a cent; by 1910, it had increased to 0.5 cents per inhabitant. Of the national budget in 1878, only 0.02 per cent was invested in health, and by 1910, the percentage had only increased to 0.54.[59]

It is important to stress that the members of the Superior Sanitation Council regarded their activities as the outcome of an apolitical observation and surveillance: "Political struggles are completely foreign to the Council, its only concern is its important and elevated mission, and it will never descend to engage its attention in political issues."[60] However, their constant surveillance and intervention was political in the sense that their actions and recommendations within the private and public life of the city's inhabitants cannot be understood as something purely altruistic or charitable. Economic, moral and public order considerations were involved, not only scientific, medical or hygienic concerns. Science, medicine and hygiene are not apolitical. Nancy Leys Stepan has pointed out that "in the history of natural sciences, issues that are social and political in character get 'scientized' (to use an ugly neologism) so that they may claim an apolitical identity from which are later drawn highly political conclusions that have considerable authority precisely because they are based on apparently neutral knowledge."[61] Following this reference to the political nature of science, it can be seen that in Mexico City, it was precisely through legislation, sanitary codes, standards for building homes, streets, markets and cemeteries, and recommendations on what were the healthy ways of living, that the various commissions that comprised the Superior Sanitation Council and the government attempted to make the urban space (with its inhabitants) an ordered and productive one. However, the actual urban transformations were neither uniform nor had the power to order urban space or make it hygienic and modern.

The Memoirs of the Sanitary Inspectors

The memoirs of the eight sanitary inspectors who belonged to the Superior Sanitation Council consisted of the reports drawn up by the commissions into which the SCC was subdivided, and of the information each sanitary inspector had gathered. Each inspector had to examine every aspect of the area under his jurisdiction and identify any unsanitary, unhealthy or hazardous conditions that required the immediate intervention of doctors, engineers and the government. [62] After 1880, the memoirs were organized following a uniform questionnaire. They all began by presenting information on various issues, placed under the heading "Diverse Documents," followed by the "Reports of the Sanitary Inspectors," and finally those of the municipalities. The report on the *cuartel* or district began by presenting neutral, objective and scientifically structured information — statistics — about the specific area under study.[63] What followed was a detailed description of all the unsanitary elements found. This generally included matters such as stagnant water; the availability of drinking water; the cleansing of streets; open sewers; open drinking water deposits and whether they were contaminated or not; the presence of litter and waste; epidemic and non-epidemic diseases encountered; the number of people vaccinated against smallpox and, after 1888, against rabies.[64] The sanitary inspectors also mentioned or detailed the positive improvements observed, as well as the measures they considered necessary to achieve a better standard of public health. However, it should be made clear that when the sanitary inspectors attempted to establish the main causes of premature death or disease, they often treated their presence in an imprecise manner. This was because there was no predominant theory for explaining disease during this period of transition between the full acceptance of the concept of microbes and germs and the gradual discrediting of the environmental theory of miasmas. According to Dr. Eduard Liceaga, the first formal clash between the defenders of the concept of miasmas and those who believed in pathogenic microbes and germs took place in 1876 during the First National Congress of Physicians. At this conference, the issues dealt with included the analysis of the unsanitary situation of the valley and city of Mexico: the lack of drinking water, the sanitary problems caused by the lack of an adequate drainage and sewer system, and the need to drain Lake Texcoco, among others.[65] It was during the discussions of these issues that opposing points of view emerged regarding how disease was spread.[66] It is therefore not surprising to find in the reports a constant aversion to mud, dust and stagnant water, while reference to germs and microbes was also made. Thus, while some doctors gradually accepted that it was germs and microbes that spread disease, others continued to attribute disease to the presence of miasmas. In some cases the two theories merged, and reference would be made to germs and microbes, while blame was also attached to the dispersion of miasmas from unsanitary areas on air currents, or to the emanation of miasmas from the land.

The Diagnoses of the City

In 1883, Dr. Ildefonso Velasco, who was then president of the Superior Sanitation Council, argued that during that year alone 13,221 people had died prematurely, and that most of those deaths had been caused by contagious diseases. The fear of contagion and the possibility of death due to the spread of disease was widespread. In 1884, the city was swept by a typhus epidemic, and in 1885, in an attempt to prevent a cholera epidemic from spreading throughout the capital, the SCC expressed that "all citizens regardless of their social standing, have an interest in this matter, and we believe that all will attempt to obey the sanitary prescriptions and to propagate the pertinent information to all social classes."[67]

In 1893, Dr. Domingo Orvañanos considered that the following epidemic diseases caused the largest numbers of premature death in Mexico City: cholera, smallpox, scarlet fever, typhus, pneumonia and diarrhoea, and that the endemic diseases were: typhus, malaria, rheumatism, smallpox, measles, scarlet fever, whooping cough and pneumonia.[68] Respiratory diseases such as tuberculosis, pneumonia and bronchitis and digestive disorders such as dysentery and diarrhoea caused the largest number of premature deaths. Respiratory diseases were widespread due to the lack of adequate housing, as was the tubercle bacillus — responsible for tuberculosis — easily spread due to the unsanitary and often overcrowded housing. The main source of diseases of the digestive system was the lack of clean water and proper sanitation throughout the city. Cholera and typhoid fever are also water-borne maladies, and conditions within the city favoured their presence and propagation. Infant mortality was predominantly caused by the highly contagious measles, scarlet fever and smallpox.[69] However, among the most feared diseases was typhus, or *tabardillo mexicano*, which was highly contagious and transmitted by lice, rat fleas and mites, and which prevailed in overcrowded unsanitary conditions. Between 1900 and 1909, the registered number of people who died prematurely in Mexico City was 28,686, as Table 3 shows.

While most diseases were explained as resulting from corrupted air and impure water, the inclusion of germs into studies of the origin and spread of disease led to the expansion of the schema of possible dangers and reinforced the association between dirt and disease. Mexican doctors of the late nineteenth century became alert to a host of new dangers — invisible to man — but present throughout the city, in all homes and all rooms. Therefore, not only was the city pathologized, but each and every house and individual was considered a latent threat.

The Capital of the nation was described as the most unsanitary and dirty city in the entire world. Thus, on the one hand, there was a genuine medical concern, and on the other, one that had more to do with the image the Capital had. And indeed, the image of the city was constantly undermined by a range of factors. Most streets had no pavement, and when it rained the streets became rivers of mud. In the centre of the city most streets were paved, but during the rainy season they often became shallow canals. Water was not the only element that made the city a foul-smelling and dangerous place. Some public markets were well known for their unsanitary conditions — Santa Catarina, Volador, San Lucas and Baratillo — among them. It was not unusual to find large amounts of litter on the streets and, occasionally, dead animals that remained exposed for days until the waste collection and disposal service arrived.[70]

Table 3: Number of premature deaths in Mexico City, 1900–09.

	Typhoid fever	Typhus	Smallpox	Measles	Scarlet fever	Whooping cough	Diphtheria and croup	Yellow fever	Erysipelas	Tuberculosis	Septicaemia
1900	16	461	345	39	21	51	21	5	102	1155	77
1901	46	1379	12	449	14	150	28	0	201	1345	79
1902	50	1338	45	58	14	157	18	7	113	1325	53
1903	29	515	216	131	36	80	31	4	89	1138	53
1904	30	248	102	99	33	132	52	0	63	1125	59
1905	27	389	157	134	8	158	70	1	124	1159	85
1906	34	1230	549	25	20	121	67	0	112	1169	93
1907	27	485	383	203	16	85	82	0	93	1157	92
1908	29	743	465	88	379	143	167	0	74	1275	75
1909	35	583	544	148	453	109	129	0	121	1210	104
Total	323	7371	2818	1374	994	1186	665	17	1092	12058	788

Source: "Anexo número 13," in *La salubridad é higiene pública en los Estados Unidos Mexicanos: Brevísima reseña de los progresos alcanzados desde 1810 hasta 1910. Publicada por el Consejo Superior de Salubridad, bajo cuyos auspicios tuvo á bien poner la Secretaría de Estado y del Despacho de Gobernación las Conferencias y la Exposición Popular de Higiene, con las cuales se sirvió contribuir a la celebración del Primer Centenario de la Independencia Nacional. Año del Centenario, 1910* (Mexico City: Casa Metodista de Publicaciones, 1910), n.p.

Many people had to sleep on the streets due to the lack of housing, and those who did have a home often lived in crowded conditions in buildings that were old and badly built or preserved. Much of the population was engaged in street commerce, selling fruit, cooked food, raw meat and fruit-flavoured water on street corners. This commerce could not function in remotely hygienic conditions, and the vendors had no licence to sell products and paid no taxes. And if all that were not enough, the city was plagued with *pulquerías* "whose absurd names underscored the contrast with the 'civilized' world."[71]

During the late nineteenth century, the high level of alcoholism among the urban population led some prominent figures, such as Julio Guerrero, to state that alcoholism caused the degeneration of the Mexican race and increased the crime rate.[72] In 1901, there were 946 *pulquerías* open during the day and 365 open only in the evening, that is, there was one *pulquería* per 307 inhabitants and, by contrast, only 34 bakeries, one bakery per 30 *pulquerías*, and 321 butchers, one per thousand inhabitants.[73] Some public health officials argued that the owners of *pulquerías* should not be forced to install public toilets, because the efficient functioning and thorough cleanliness required would never be maintained due to their uneducated public.[74] For the Porfirian elite, all the elements so far mentioned were considered detrimental both to the image of the modern city and to the general well-being of the population. In 1899, the newspaper *El Mundo* stressed that the image of the modern city was constantly shattered by the presence of elements such as narrow, dirty and foul-smelling cul-de-sacs, street vendors and tenement buildings.[75]

Another major problem was that the social behaviour, customs and practices of the majority of the population were regarded as inappropriate to a clean and modern city. What particularly worried the members of the Superior Sanitation Council was the lack of cleanliness of the urban population. Not only was the city filthy, but most of its inhabitants were seen as dirty and as possible carriers of some sort of disease. Thus, the dirtiness of the city was equated by public health officials and foreigners alike with the dirtiness of the people. Protestant Anglo-American travelers often described the country and its people as primitive and backward, and portrayed the Mexican people as "a weak, effete, mongrel, withered race," added remarks about the lack of cleanliness and wondered how the Mexican people could "survive so long in unwholesome conditions."[76]

Both the independent national press, and that subsidized by the government, referred to the dirtiness of the streets, to the infected air the inhabitants were forced to breathe, and to the tainted water of its remaining canals. In guides to the city, written by both foreign and national travelers, it was emphasized that in spite of the erection of impressive public buildings and monuments, the dirtiness of its people destroyed the "modern" atmosphere, reminding travelers — and also a minority of Mexicans — that they were indeed not in Paris or London, but in Mexico City.

In addition, bathing was said to be a rare experience among the urban poor: at the turn of the century there was one public bathhouse per fifteen thousand inhabitants.[77] However, there was one day of the year that was seen by many national and foreign observers as a miraculous date: 24 June, the day of Saint John the Baptist, when, according to the tradition of the festival, most Mexicans bathed. However, on that day, bathing was seen as being the result of religious ritual rather than of the science of hygiene.[78]

Another major health hazard was the adulteration of food: bakeries sold biscuits leavened with lead chromate; milk was regularly diluted with dirty water and thickened with animal brains discarded by the slaughterhouses and butchers; cat or dog meat were sold as beef; and often coffee was mixed with chickpeas and bread crumbs.[79]

The various commissions of the Superior Sanitation Council were aware of these problems, as well as of the overcrowded and unsanitary conditions that prevailed not only in popular housing but also in jails and hospitals. For instance, the Epidemics Commission placed special emphasis on preventing the spread of diseases such as cholera, yellow fever, tuberculosis, typhus and smallpox in hospitals, prisons, and other places of confinement.[80] This commission worked closely with the vaccination commission; in 1888, the *Instituto Antirrábico* was created, and between 1888 and 1891 407 people were vaccinated against rabies.

In addition, a free service for the diagnosis of tuberculosis and typhoid fever was set up, and between 1900 and 1904, 12,735 homes were disinfected, as well as 19,288 rooms and 179,342 items of clothing belonging to people who had been in contact with or had had typhus, yellow fever or tuberculosis.[81] However, in 1905, after a typhus epidemic, the health authorities issued a set of sanitary measures to be adhered to by the urban population. And once more, the emphasis was on ordering the people to clean the city, their homes, themselves, and to change their habits and day-to-day practices.[82] Some measures dealt specifically with the enforcement of precise legislation governing the activities of the urban population. Other measures involved the provision of public services and basic urban infrastructure. Yet others implied a more thorough degree of control over, or intrusion of the medical profession into, the lives and social practices of the poorest sectors of the urban population; for instance, people were taken to the police station and forced to bathe, and beggars were removed from the city's streets.

Overcrowding was regarded as one of the main elements that contributed to the presence and spread of disease. In 1882, the journal of the Municipal Council, *El Municipio Libre*, published a detailed report on the measures that had to be taken by everyone in order to avoid succumbing to cholera, and the emphasis was placed on avoiding large gatherings and overcrowding wherever possible.[83]

In 1895, Dr. Domingo Orvañanos referred to the horrible and disgusting promiscuity and dangerous social consequences that could be observed in tenement buildings due to overcrowding. According to him, more than a hundred thousand people lived in tenement buildings where humidity, darkness and filth prevailed.[84] In addition, because pollution and contagion often began in the home, the individual body was regarded as a potential pollutant, and therefore overcrowding had to be avoided. Of particular concern were the dwellings of the poor, because they were said to be a source of epidemic disease and to constitute a threat to the well-being and health of all social classes.[85] In 1901, the report of Vicente Montes de Oca, sanitary inspector of the Second Quarter, considered the housing problems in this area of the city to be serious due to the number of inhabitants — 70,239.[86] He suggested that in order to avoid overcrowding in buildings and homes, it was necessary to build hygienic, cheap and segregated housing for the proletarians.[87]

The threat posed by overcrowding was also pointed out by Dr. Bernáldez, sanitary inspector of the Sixth Quarter, who stated that it was imperative to prevent excessive proximity of people — five, six or more people sharing a room. He also considered that certain material elements of all dwellings had to be modified; for instance, he suggested that they had to possess paved floors and bathrooms, and explicitly asserted that no one should have animals inside the household.[88] The presence of roaming animals inside the homes within the city represented a threat to health and blurred the distinction between city and countryside which the Porfirian elite was eager to impose upon the capital.

Doctor Bernáldez also suggested that clothes should not be left to dry in the *patios* but in the *azoteas*, because the sight of them at the entrance or on the top floor of a tenement building or home was not pleasant, and also because in the *patios* the airborne miasmas would be more easily inhaled by people.[89] But above all, the recommendations aimed to transform the working and social practices of the urban population and to attain a marked segregation of functions inside the private space — the home. The aim was to make space — be it private or public — segregated, giving each activity a specially designated site. This segregation of activities was to affect the entire city.[90]

Health considerations went far beyond the realm of public health and became an instrument through which, in the name of the collective health of the city, public health officials aimed to alter the private lives, practices, customs and behaviour of the urban population. Thus, when physicians and hygienists considered questions of order and health, the realms of morality, disease and crime easily overlapped. In order to restrain the development of disease, it was necessary to ensure that the recommendations made by the Superior Sanitation Council were followed by all the urban population, but particularly by the slum-dwelling poor. What took place within private space — the home — was continually checked by public health officials, and all streets and public spaces were also subject to constant laws and regulation.[91]

In 1905, the sanitary inspector of the Third Quarter, Dr. Manuel Soriano, began his report by reflecting on the difficulties and problems responsible citizens like himself continuously encountered in the battle for a clean and decent capital. Although his ideas are detailed, it is important to quote him at length, because they sum up the notions held at the time by public health officials, and show how their mission was associated with or defined as a war:

> The application of hygiene in our country has hardly begun, and the labor which the Council has been doing since it was created is arduous, almost verging on the unbelievable, given that our Capital inherited from our ancestors all the vices of organization

in the home, in the streets and in the dwellings; given that the destitute take little care of themselves, of their family and relatives around them. Through its popular publications, by corrective measures, by persuasion, by entreaty, perhaps finally by violence, the Council has wanted to impose the means to preserve health, to prevent disease, to give to the country hereafter healthy and strong individuals who can serve their families in the home, their fellow men in society, their country, in short, defending their country when it is attacked, and when not, working ceaselessly for its advancement and progress, and to achieve this desired goal, there is public and private hygiene.[92]

According to Soriano, the struggle was against all kinds of obstacles, some moral, others physical, and some even hereditary. The members of the Superior Sanitation Council had tried to correct the bad habits of the people through all sorts of procedures, through education or even violence when necessary. The idea of having healthy people who benefit the nation and its economic progress is clearly spelled out by this inspector, as well as the role assumed by public health officials of instigating a thorough hygienic and moral reform of the Mexican people. Alan Knight has pointed out that during the Porfiriato much stress was laid on the "inherent defects of 'the people,'" and that if solutions were sought at all, "they often belonged to the realm of education and propaganda, which might complement the old resort to coercion."[93]

However, a serious problem the city faced was the lack of an abundant supply of drinking water, a problem that persists to this day. Manuel Soriano mentioned that the lack of water was particularly worrying, and that twenty-four streets in the Third Quarter had no water at all, and although he knew that 102 wells were in operation at various points, their conditions were defined as being far from adequate.[94] Many public wells throughout the city were infected by cesspool seepage and not maintained at all, and they were a real threat to the health of those who drank or cooked with the water. It was widely believed, as Soriano pointed out, that the cleansing of the streets with this water was a sure way to spread disease. The two main diseases in the Third Quarter of the city were typhus and smallpox. The total number of people reported to have had typhus was 145: sixty-nine male and seventy-six female, and Soriano explained the causes as follows:

From sunstroke, 7 cases; from contagion, 16 cases; from cold, 38 cases; from damp, 16 cases; from infection, 53 cases and in 15 cases the cause is unknown. From this small picture it can be deduced that infection and cold make up the largest contingent: the first is impregnated in those who are poverty-stricken ..., and the latter from the lack of shelter and heat in the dwellings.[95]

Soriano considered that the highest incidence of typhus was found among the urban poor, and that from there it could extend to all social classes. Not only were the causes of typhus confusing, but the wish to blame the possible spread of typhus on the poor shows how a specific sector of the urban population was thought to be a source of disease. For Soriano, epidemics always began in the dwellings of the poor because they paid little or no attention to the principles of private and public hygiene. [96] Persuasion and even threats were the weapons that hygienists employed against the social practices of the city's population, and physicians hoped that future generations would transform their habits and customs through education.[97]

The expansion of the city, as has been mentioned, was enhanced by the construction of a communications infrastructure, including rail tracks, which created internal divisions within the capital. Doctor Salvador Quevedo y Zubieta, the sanitary inspector of the Seventh Quarter, was of the opinion that the expansion of the city in this area had produced very contrasting results. This quarter was made up of two main sections, one to the east and the other to the west. This clear-cut division created by the stations, offices and rail tracks of the Ferrocarriles Centrales and Mexicano, was described as follows by Quevedo y Zubieta:

> These areas differ much from the hygienist point of view. In the east — the *colonia* Guerrero — the population is denser and poorer than in the west (the *colonias* San Cosme and Santa María). In the east there are many tenements that with their human crowds in sombre, damp and badly ventilated hovels seem to be constantly defying Sanitation and its Superior Council, however much they are subjected to repeated inspections. In the west private houses with modern constructions prevail, in which hygienic conditions are more feasible. Nevertheless, among them there are many remains of the old collective kind of housing and toward the boundaries of the colonia Santa María

the provisional houses awaiting reconstruction multiply, the divided-up properties, some inhabited by tenants, others by wardens, all living in a primitive way in the company of the farmyard animals that are reared there.[98]

The above statement shows how within the same quarter some *colonias* had better services and housing than others, indicating the segregation of the population along economic lines. The agent of division between the eastern and western areas of this quarter was the railroad. The rail tracks invading the city led to the erection of physical barriers in areas of the city that until then had had no internal borders. The sanitary inspector also mentioned that many *barrios* or *pueblecitos extra-muros* existed, and named San Miguel Nonoalco and Atlampa. He stated that because these *barrios* were outside what was considered to be the urban perimeter, they had no access to the drinking water or sewers that areas "inside" the city had or should have. The *publecitos extra-muros* were defined as "total barbarism at the threshold of our incipient culture of hygiene."[99] The threat of backwardness and filth was just at the city gates. Sarmiento in Argentina had referred to the desert that surrounded the city as a latent threat; in Mexico City, the threat was identified with the regions that remained at the margins of the modern city.

Quevedo y Zubieta also recommended bridging the divide created by the railway tracks, a division that was detrimental to the prosperity of the entire area, and attacked the disruption and chaos brought about by the railways, the symbol of economic progress. He suggested that the task of solving the problems created by the rail tracks fell to the engineer, and that the hygienist simply made general recommendations.[100] However, during this period, engineers, physicians and hygienists worked very closely together, and on most occasions it was the public works carried out by engineers that fulfilled the demands made by public health officials.

The images of the city presented by public health officials were as important as statistics, and the numbers of people who were ill or had died were used to give authority to their observations. The careful and constant observation of the city was at the core of public health officials' activities, and these studies, as has been shown, tried to be more than mere descriptions, more than naturalist snapshots of the capital. Through them the officials aimed to present the problems and propose possible solutions. However, the studies revealed truly deplorable situations, and the language used in them was generally rich in adjectives and moral undertones. They managed to shock the reader, to influence public opinion and aimed to highlight social pathologies of the social organism (of society). They were persuasive and aroused concern, and public health officials believed that their research was carried out according to scientific procedures and rules.

The image of the modern city, seen through medical eyes, had to be clean and odourless and free from visible overcrowding, conditions which assumed the thorough observation and classification of most activities taking place in the city. Through the reports or memoirs of the Superior Sanitation Council, it has been possible to see how the city looked, and how it *had* to look, and why so many different aspects of urban life were taken into consideration. The city had to have a degree of uniformity in its appearance and in its functioning. To this end, public health officials contributed their knowledge by pinpointing everything that was wrong; engineers contributed their plans and projects for public works, public buildings and monuments; architects and artists, their sculptures and other works of art; foreigners, their capital and engineering expertise.

An important achievement for the modern city was the ability to control epidemic disease and contagious illnesses. The impact that contagious diseases, and in particular epidemic outbreaks, had on the city was widespread, and it involved all the population in some way or another: succumbing to disease, having a member of the family, a friend or an acquaintance who was ill; being unable to work or socialize. It also stigmatized the diseased individual, in particular if he/she was poor. This period was one when the association between disease and dirt was firmly established and when it fully permeated the discourse of physicians and hygienists. Both dirt and disease were dangerous elements that had to be eradicated or placed under control. A healthy urban population was indispensable for the economy and meant that the productive process was unaffected by disease. However, the reports submitted by the sanitary inspectors show that it was believed that ignorance, lack of morality and carelessness within the majority of the urban population constituted the main obstacles to attaining a truly hygienic city. It was thought that through education, many of the social customs would change and that once people adhered to hygienic principles, the city would benefit enormously. It was not enough for doctors to identify the hazards encountered; it was necessary to educate the people, to cultivate in them a "hygienic instinct" based on science, rather than superstition or religion.[101]

So far, this study has not dealt with the deliberate changes to the physiognomy of the city, such as the erection of public buildings and monuments, or the architectural styles adopted in specific *colonias*, or the importance of new systems of terrestrial communication, in terms of the overall functioning of the city. Neither has it examined the importance of monuments to the image of the modern city. Instead it has attempted to present the aspects of Mexico City that were incompatible with this image. However, a key aspect of Porfirian Mexico City was the establishment of a correspondence between the urban landscape and the image of order and progress that the elite had forged of itself.[102]

Therefore, the next chapter will examine how specific areas of the city were deliberately transformed by the construction of public buildings and monuments. It will examine how this localized urban design was inspired by the model of European capital cities, such as Paris and London, and how the Porfirian elite thought of a modern city as a clean and monumental one. The symbolic significance of the city as a centre of political and economic power, order and culture led some sectors of the urban population to consider its expansion as tangible and visible proof of the era of order and progress in which they were living. On 9 August 1887, the editorial of *El Municipio Libre* was proud to state that, for some time

> we have observed with satisfaction, that in the accounts that are published about travels to Mexico, and in particular to the Capital of the Republic, those passionate and unjust appraisals have ceased, inspired only by the impression of the moment, and which made us look like as savage nation, living in towns bereft of all that which forms the basis of comfort and culture.[103]

How that modernity, culture and cleanliness was built into a city that the Porfirian regime was eager to display to nationals and foreigners alike will be explored in the following chapter.

4

The Modern City

The unsanitary conditions in the capital and the unfavourable geographic location on which it was built led to the exacerbation of public health problems, to thorough surveys of the city, and to numerous laws and regulations that aimed to cleanse the city and keep it ordered and hygienic throughout the year. The image of the modern city required cleanliness and hygiene, but it was also important to display the modernization of the country, its political stability and the progress achieved in the arts, industry and science. The best way to do this was by building monuments to honour the men and the heroic actions that had been important in the formation of the nation, and to this end, numerous statues and monuments were unveiled by the government. In 1892, the newspaper *El Universal* stated that the mania for erecting statues was acquiring epidemic proportions.[1] Public space was being modernized.

The attempt to transform the appearance of the city and endow it with prestige and originality led to the deliberate altering of the urban landscape on specific sites. The prime site was the new locus of power that traversed the modern city, the Paseo de la Reforma. This chapter will look at public space not as a neutral site, but as a site "embedded with politics and ideology, both real and imagined, which afford space with the contextualisation of power."[2] Through the construction of monuments, the modern city became the site where the symbols of power were displayed and reinforced, and monuments were regarded not only as concrete representations of the nation and of its modernity, but also as vehicles for the education of the Mexican people. Additionally, monumental space, as well as avenues, plazas and gardens, became identified as areas that would promote the relaxation, morally suitable amusement, hygiene and health of the city's inhabitants.

Towards the Secular City

The expansion of the city began during the late 1850s and 1860s and led to profound changes following the secularization of urban property. The Lerdo Law (issued by Miguel Lerdo de Tejada in 1856) and the Laws of Reform (issued by Benito Juárez, 7 July 1859) decreed the suppression of communal Indian landholdings as well as the restriction of ecclesiastical rights over private ownership. When this law came into force in 1861, the Church's wealth was valued at approximately 150 million pesos.[3] Many ecclesiastical buildings were re-utilized by the state for non-religious purposes, and churches, convents and hospitals were employed as schools, municipal and government buildings, public offices, museums and libraries. The aim was to transform the city into a secular city and to imprint upon public space the power of the secular state. However, due to lack of resources and political instability throughout most of the second half of the nineteenth century, the construction of new buildings, both by the government and by private individuals, was very limited. The only architectural genre that did not decline throughout the century was funerary architecture.[4] The uninterrupted construction of tombs and the re-utilization of ecclesiastical buildings were accompanied by the demolishing of churches and convents as the century advanced.

The secularization of urban property and land was part of an attempt to forge a national identity within the urban landscape, and the secularization of cultural expressions led to a search for historical heroes and events that would legitimize the emergence of the liberal, secular and independent nation-state. In Mexico City, the religious names of streets and plazas gradually gave way to civilian names ratifying those in power or those who had made possible the separation between Church and state. Religious festivals and celebrations were also gradually supplemented by others that had a more civic character. Public sites such as avenues, parks and plazas became the places where these celebrations would take place and where the monuments that narrated the national, secular and official version of Mexico's history would stand.

The deliberate use of public space to reaffirm the nation did not begin during the Porfiriato, but it was then when secular and national symbols of Mexico as an independent and modern nation were erected in the capital. Before the final decades of the nineteenth century, there were numerous attempts to secularize public space and to reinforce the idea of the nation, and not only were convents and churches demolished, but plans and projects were submitted to create monuments, statues and other symbols representing the nation.[5] In 1862, for instance, the government decided to commemorate its triumph against the French in Puebla during the battle of 5 May by establishing that date as a national festival, and it also planned to erect two monumental fountains in the Alameda. One of the fountains was to be named "5th of May" Fountain.[6] The enthusiasm following Mexico's victory in the Battle of Puebla was short-lived, and during the French Empire (1864–67), Emperor Maximilian attempted to strengthen his reign and to gain supporters through the construction of public monuments, by remodelling certain areas of the city as well as the Castle of Chapultepec, the Imperial residence.[7] He also commissioned artists to paint large historical works, and Santiago Rebull undertook a series of portraits of the heroes of Independence, including Hidalgo, Morelos and Iturbide. On 14 June 1864, Maximilian expressed his wish to build a monument to Mexico's Independence. The first stone was placed upon the Plaza Mayor, or Zócalo, by his wife Carlota on 16 September 1864. However, this project was abandoned and a new competition was publicized in September 1865.[8]

By November it was known that the competition had been won by engineer Ramón Rodríguez Arangoity, but his project was abandoned, and manpower and resources from the Ministry of Development, through its Departamento de Inspección de Caminos, were allocated for the construction and repair of streets, avenues, bridges, and for the long-awaited drainage system for the city. It was also during the French Empire that the Paseo del Emperador (renamed Paseo de la Reforma in 1872) was built, a site selected by the Porfirian regime to become the visible centre of the country.

The construction of the Paseo del Emperador began in 1864 and was concluded the following year. It was built in response to the need for an adequate means of communication between the Castle of Chapultepec and the centre of the city. The new boulevard ran in a straight line from the castle to the statue of

Charles IV, and was built for the personal use of the Emperor by the urban developer Francisco Somera.[9] The Paseo had a length of 3,435 metres and a width of eighteen metres, and each pavement was nine metres wide. The source of inspiration for this *paseo*, or boulevard, has been attributed to the boulevards in Paris constructed under Emperor Napoleon III by the Prefect of Paris, George Eugène Haussmann.[10] It has also been stated that Maximilian was influenced by the urban reforms initiated in Austria by his brother, the Emperor Franz Josef, and in particular by the construction of the Ringstrasse in Vienna, which replaced the encircling walls of the Austrian capital.[11] Leaving aside the question of whether what influenced Maximilian was the French or the Austrian example, what must be stressed is that the construction of this avenue was not part of a thorough or comprehensive urban design, as was the case with the urban reforms of Paris. The construction of the Paseo del Emperador was carried out to solve a practical problem, as there was no adequate road linking the Imperial residence and the centre of the city. This new axis of communication had important implications for the future expansion of the city. The symbolic importance of the central district of the city throughout its history was shifted to this new site during the Porfiriato. The expansion and direction of the city followed its course, and so did real estate speculation and construction. The modern city was built along and across this boulevard, and this area served the purpose of giving the upper middle classes a place in which to assert their cultural and economic identity apart from the people at large, particularly the indigenous and poor sectors of the urban population.[12]

After the Restoration of the Republic in 1867, the Paseo del Emperador was renamed Calzada Degollado, and on 19 February 1872, Benito Juárez changed its name to Paseo de la Reforma and declared it to be for the use of all citizens, whether on foot, horse or any other means of transport. By 1872, the Paseo de la Reforma's dimensions were almost the same as they had been in 1866: 3,460 metres in length, eighteen metres in width for animal-drawn vehicles and nine metres on each pavement for pedestrians. It also had numerous trees, including 486 willows and seventeen ash trees. During the presidency of Sebastián Lerdo de Tejada (1872–76), more trees were planted on its pavements, benches were set out for the relaxation of visitors, the president encouraged civic leaders to formulate plans for its beautification, and a monument to Cristóbal Colón was donated by railroad entrepreneur Antonio Escandón in 1873 to commemorate the opening of his railroad to Veracruz that same year.[13] This monument was erected and unveiled on the Paseo de la Reforma in 1877.

To walk along the Paseo during the last years of the Porfiriato constituted an educational experience, as historical monuments were placed along the *glorietas* and on the pavement of this long avenue. Many homes also adopted architectural styles not seen before in the city, and the visual changes in the capital were greeted as tangible evidence of the modernity of the country. Before examining these monuments, their purpose and symbolic meaning, the next section will briefly explore how the modernity of the city was highlighted by looking at some of the descriptions of it written during the Porfiriato.

The Image of the Modern City

During the last decades of the nineteenth century and from 1900 to 1910, numerous accounts were written by Mexicans and foreigners commenting on the material progress that was being achieved in the capital city.[14] Some descriptions approached the city from a bird's-eye view, narrowing the focus as the gaze descended to a key site; others would approach the city from the outskirts, from the countryside to the suburbs and from there to the centre, where the Cathedral and Plaza Mayor stood. Constant emphasis was placed on its modern aspect, the importance of the physical changes brought about since Porfirio Díaz had been in power. In guides to the city, everything was reviewed: its streets, canals, avenues, railway tracks, railway stations, government buildings, industries, days of celebration (religious or secular), schools, markets, theatres, sports, professions, dress, food; many were accompanied by maps, illustrations, engravings, photographs and *cartes de visite*.[15] While the detailed review of some of the elements mentioned above could not omit reference to the inhabitants of the city, or to the numerous setbacks the modernizing project in fact had suffered, such as the eternal flooding of the city, many photographs and illustrations accompanying the texts presented views of an uninhabited city.[16] The emphasis was placed on its avenues, buildings, railways stations and monuments; in other words, stress was placed on capturing the evidence of progress.[17]

Adolfo Prantl and José Groso defined the city in 1901 as uninhabited, as a city formed by a multiplicity of fragments as described in the following words:

> In the same way as looking through the lens of a kaleidoscope, the following is seen when viewing the city: high and low roofs, shop signs, fragments of fa ades, many-colored walls, bright passageways with flowerpots of geraniums, roses, jasmine and heliotropes, high windows with thin white curtains, large green patches — our gardens that embalm the atmosphere — , windmills, towers, water tanks, and in short, a motley coloring of many things ... and afterwards ... a very extensive plain which surrounds the city and in which the lakes of Texcoco, Chalco and Xochimilco and the canals of the Viga and of San Lázaro shine like glittering mirrors.[18]

This fragmented perception of the city presented an image of constant visual change, and all the foul-smelling water of Lake Texcoco, and indeed that within the city, simply did not exist. Neither its people nor its sanitary problems were mentioned. By the turn of the century, it was still possible to see the whole of the city from above. Some photographs taken during the last two decades of the nineteenth century and the beginning of this century by Guillermo Kahlo and Hugo Brehme show that the central part of the city could be traversed and explored on foot and that most *colonias* could be reached by the use of streetcars. In the city's centre, most buildings were of a uniform height, that is, most were no taller than three or four floors, some had balconies that looked out on the streets, the roofs were flat, and the only visual elements that stood out among the buildings were the towers of the churches and of the Cathedral. From the roof of any three- or four-storey building, the mountains encircling the valley could be clearly seen, and even at ground level they could be seen on the horizon.

Some photographs also showed that some areas were undergoing profound changes, causing disruption to the day-to-day activities of the population. The construction of new public and governmental buildings, large commercial stores and an underground system of sewers and drainage made sectors of the city look like huge building sites. Everyday activities taking place in the numerous open markets, the traffic of the street vendors and water carriers, and of bureaucrats going from one office to another, coexisted with the work of the numerous builders, architects, engineers and physicians who supervised the construction of public works and buildings. The sounds of church bells were accompanied by the sounds street vendors, trains, machines and the large number of workers who operated them.

The most exclusive and fashionable *colonias* were located along both sides of the Paseo de la Reforma. They were the *colonias* La Teja, Paseo, Americana, Nueva del Paseo, Juárez, Cuauhtémoc, Roma and Condesa. The land on which the *colonia* Cuauhtémoc was built had been bought and divided from the Hacienda de la Teja (its original name having been Stilwell Place, but changed to *colonia* Cuauhtémoc to honour the memory of the last Aztec emperor).[19] This area of the city gradually came to acquire most public services, such as drinking water and sewers, and its paved streets were named Roma, Milán, Lucerna, Dinamarca, Hamburgo, Londres, Berlín and Amazonas. The *colonia* Roma was built following the French urban model of mid-nineteenth century Paris, which stressed the presence of wide avenues (boulevards), *étoiles*, fountains and well-kept gardens. The *colonia* Condesa was built on land that had belonged to the Hacienda de la Condesa and linked the city to the municipality of Tacubaya.

Photographs also allowed the families living in the modern city to display their lifestyle and sense of well-being. Photographs of interiors emphasized material possessions, and the Mexicans and foreigners who lived in the most prestigious *colonias* imported all sorts of furniture and prefabricated decorative elements, such as lamps, pianos, furniture, carpets, curtains, paintings, marble and/or bronze statues, fountains, silver and glass.[20] Many houses in the modern *colonias* displayed a range of architectural styles, and according to Israel Katzman the predominant style was eclecticism.[21] The multiplicity of architectural styles and materials accompanying the construction fever that swept across some areas of the capital can be appreciated by briefly examining some of them.

From the 1870s onward, plans were drawn up for railway stations in the city, and many began to adopt the use of visible iron for their structures. Iron was also used to make street lamps and benches in parks and gardens, and for the construction of kiosks in central plazas and private gardens. In 1878, an iron kiosk was placed in the centre of the Plaza Mayor or Zócalo, and from that date many squares in other cities began to adopt the same fashion. The use of iron also made it possible to construct taller buildings and to support monuments. The first building to be entirely built with iron structures was the Centro Mercantil (1896–97). Another building that incorporated iron into its structure was the department store El Palacio de Hierro (1889), as well as the Teatro Nacional (Palacio de Bellas Artes), the Palacio Legislativo (which became the Monumento a la Revolución), the Edificio de Correos and the building of the Secretaría de Comunicaciones, all begun between 1900 and 1910. Some architects and engineers also began to adopt the fashion of building homes with mansard roofs, as in the case of the house of the Braniff family on the Paseo de la Reforma, built in 1888 by the English architect Charles S. Hall. Between 1890 and 1900, this style was also used in other houses, including the house of José Yves Limantour, in the jewel store La Esmeralda, in commercial buildings and in the roof of the railway station Interocéanico. Other styles that made their presence felt in the city were the Neo-Gothic, such as the Edificio Central de Correos built by the Italian architect Adamo Boari (1902–06), as well as the Baroque, the Muslim, Art Nouveau and Romantic.[22] An important innovation of the time was the use of pre-Hispanic figures and decorative elements. The Indigenista or neo pre-Hispanic style first appeared in the city with the monument to Cuauhtémoc and with the statues of the Aztec kings Ahuítzotl and Itzcóatl, all erected on the Paseo de la Reforma.

The Porfirian peace and the relative stability of the economy allowed the government to invest large amounts of capital in the material embellishment of Mexico City. The embellishment of the capital — or more precisely of specific areas of the city — sent strong messages to the Mexican people, among them that their capital was truly a modern capital of the world on the path of progress. The embellishment of the capital was also for foreign consumption, and this was ultimately linked to the need to attract and secure foreign investment. Even though the city lacked a very strong or dominant industrial establishment, it was the centre of political and economic decision making. It was also the centre of distribution of domestic production and the focus of all railway lines. The capital housed the richest sectors of Mexico's population, and therefore concentrated income, and it also contained all the banks, which produced all of the country's bank notes in 1885, and still almost two thirds of the national total in 1910. In addition, ninety-two percent of all credit was extended in the Federal District in 1890, and seventy-four percent even in 1911, after state banks had been established.[23]

Additionally, it had foreign investors, who were the prime movers behind the country's major banks. To a great extent, Mexico City's financial supremacy was at the expense of the rest of the country.[24] The resources allocated to public works and communications infrastructure between 1877 and 1910 benefited directly or indirectly the capital of the country. The total investment amounted to 1,036.9 million pesos and was distributed as follows: "286 million pesos of private funds, 667 millions of foreign companies and 83.9 millions invested by the government." Of the 286 millions of private investment, "92 were spent in Mexico City, 64 were for the rest of the country and the remaining 130 million pesos of general investments favored the Federal District."[25] Of the investment in infrastructural works by private funds, primarily foreign capital, ten million pesos were destined for the construction of electric trams in the Federal District, electricity and telephone services in Mexico City received twelve million pesos, and foreign capital for Federal banks and State banks without Federal concessions amounted to ninety million pesos.[26] With regard to the infrastructural works contracted by the government with foreign capital, Table 4 shows the importance of foreign investment for the efficient functioning of the city.

Without underestimating the industrial, financial and commercial role of the city, which has been studied in numerous books and articles,[27] and which is not the subject of this work, what must be stressed is the importance for the city of the public works marked with an asterisk in Table 4. The drainage works for the valley and city of Mexico, the public works to cleanse the city of all its stagnant water and the installation of an efficient system of underground sewers were all praised as the most important projects ever undertaken, and their conclusion would make the capital a clean and efficient example of the modernity of the nation. The investment in railway lines eased the national and international circulation of agricultural, industrial and mineral products, and converged in the capital of the nation.

The role played by foreign investors was fundamental to the material upgrading and embellishment of the capital. So just as foreign investors were allocating large sums of money for the capital, in ports and railways, the Díaz government invested in the construction of monuments and public buildings to give the capital a truly modern and solid appearance, as Table 5 shows. The total investment made by the government amounted to

Table 4: Public works undertaken by the government contracted with foreign capital, 1877–1910 (in millions of pesos)

Public work	Investment
1 Public works in the Port of Veracruz contracted with the British firm Pearson	33.0
2 Contracts with Pearson for Tehuantepec and ports	104.0
3 Drainage works for the Valley of Mexico ★	14.0
4 Construction and equipment for 18,000 km of rail tracks, federal concession ★	500.0
5 Sanitary works in the Port of Veracruz	4.0
6 Public works in the Port of Tampico	6.0
7 Sanitary works in Mexico City ★	6.0
Total	667.0

Source: Diego López Rosado. *Historia y pensamiento económico de México. Finanzas Públicas – Obras Públicas* (Mexico City: Universidad Nacional Autónoma de México, 1972), 148.

83.9 million pesos, and only 14.7 million were destined for public works and infrastructure outside Mexico City. The capital received 69.2 million pesos, that is, 82.5 per cent of the total. Of that amount, twelve million were spent on the introduction of drinking water, but the rest was invested either in the construction of impressive governmental buildings (such as the Palacio Legislativo, the Chamber of Deputies, the building of the Secretaría de Comunicaciones y Obras Públicas and the Edificio de Correos), or in the paving of the city's streets, the Gran Opera (Bellas Artes) and the monuments to Cuauhtémoc and to Independence. The Paseo de la Reforma and the Bosque de Chapultepec also received a generous share of capital. However, as Table 5 shows, not all went towards embellishing the city and upgrading its unsanitary conditions. Large sums of money were also allocated to the construction of the Penitentiary and the General Hospital, institutions that point towards the importance of creating places of confinement, control and scientific inquiry during the Porfiriato. However, both the investment made by the Federal Government and that made by foreigners benefited Mexico City directly or indirectly. The centralization of power in the capital required a city that conformed or appeared to conform to ideals of power and stability.

Table 5: Public works undertaken directly by the government, 1877–1910 (in millions of pesos).

Public Work	Investment
1 Paving of Mexico City	8.0
2 Public works for the distribution of drinking water for the capital	12.0
3 Monument to Independence in Mexico City	1.5
4 Public works for the drainage and irrigation of Chapala	2.7
5 Construction of schools in the Federal District	2.5
6 Theatre Gran Opera in Mexico City until 1911	11.0
7 Building of the Secretaría de Comunicaciones y Obras Públicas	3.8
8 Building of Correos	3.5
9 Palacio Legislativo	8.0
10 Diverse Public works	3.0
11 General Hospital and other buildings	6.0
12 New Chamber of Deputies	0.3
13 Telegraphs throughout the Republic, telephones, light-houses and Federal buildings outside the Federal District	12.0
14 Penitentiary, Ex-aduana de Santiago Tlatelolco and Monument to Cuauhtémoc	4.6
15 Cost of the expropriation of land for the Gran Opera and for the Paseo de la Reforma	4.6
16 Bosque de Chapultepec	0.4
Total	83.9

Source: Diego López Rosado. *Historia y pensamiento económico en México. Finanzas Públicas — Obras Públicas* (Mexico City: Universidad Nacional Autónoma de México, 1972), 149.

Some sectors of *capitalinos* believed that the embellishment of the city was unquestionable tangible evidence of the national prosperity and modernity brought about by the liberal government of Díaz, and that foreign observers or tourists could see for themselves the progress of the capital. Mexico City was not only the visible evidence of the material prosperity of the country; it also became an example to follow in other Mexican cities, such as Puebla and Mérida. The capital city symbolized the centralization of economic decision-making and political power, and therefore it had to set a modern, stable, ordered and prosperous example to the rest of the nation and to the outside world, the source of foreign investment.

A key visual element in the depiction of the modern city was the absence of people, as mentioned earlier, and this can be appreciated by examining some of the outdoor photographs and texts that reflected the cosmopolitan progress achieved through the city's architecture and urban vistas. A depiction of a city without inhabitants, which leads us to analyze one of the main symbols of Mexican secular monuments during the Porfiriato, is the oil on canvas, *View of the Valley of México from the Hill of Santa Isabel*, painted in 1877 by José María Velasco (see Figure 1). This landscape concentrates on the vastness of the valley of Mexico, its encircling mountains, the water of Lake Texcoco, the eternal snow covering the peaks of Popocatépetl and Iztaccíhuatl, and on the rocks and hillsides characteristic of the environment. Velasco incorporated two elements that point towards the historicist nationalism invoked at the time to strengthen the idea of Mexico as a nation. In the lower left-hand corner of the painting an eagle and a cactus appear, making clear reference to the myth of the founding of Tenochtitlán by the Aztecs in 1325, the emblem of the country.[28]

The landscape surrounding the city is presented as a conquerable area, as a region of expansion for the city, and the border between the city and the countryside is emphasized by the appropriation of the founding myth of the nation by the capital. In this painting, as in other of Velasco's works — for instance, in *Puente curvo del Ferrocarril Mexicano en la cañada de Metlac* (1881) — people are omitted. What are reinforced and enhanced are the symbols of the progress of the country, the climate of political order and social peace. Whether through photographs, writing, paintings or sculptures and monuments, this approach to the city deliberately ignored the cultural differences and social distances prevalent among the urban population, and instead exalted with enthusiasm the idea of 'nation'.

The aim of modernizing public space and endowing it with the symbols of the liberal nation led to what Carlos Monsiváis has defined as one of the most favoured activities of the Porfirian elite: the homogenization of appearances.[29] The objective was to attain a homogeneous appearance or image of modernity, and the gulf that separated the liberal *patria* from the people at large was bridged through the official cult of national heroes, public holidays and civic sanctuaries. The educational and moralizing role of public space aimed to make the urban population aware of the nation, and to teach them to show respect towards national institutions and laws.

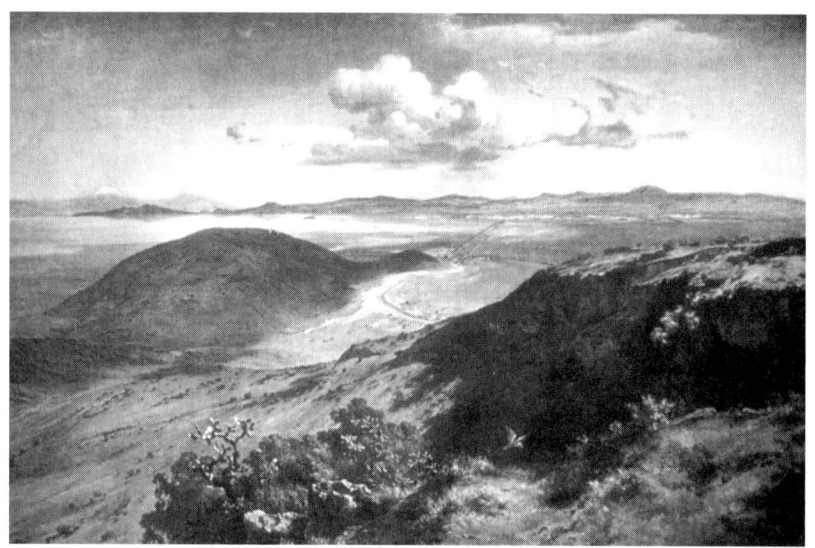

Figure 1. José María Velasco, *View of the Valley of Mexico from the Hill of Santa Isabel*, 1877, oil on canvas, 137.5 x 226 cm.
Source: Archivo Fotográfico Instituto de Investigaciones Estéticas – UNAM, Mexico City. Reproduction authorized by the Instituto Nacional de Bellas Artes y Literatura, Consejo Nacional para la Cultura y las Artes, Museo Nacional de Arte, Mexico. (Photograph by Xavier Moyssen Echeverría)

The use of Mexico's foundational or pre-Hispanic past — manifest in Velasco's pictorial incorporation of national historical elements or founding myths such as the cactus and the eagle — also featured in sculpture and architecture in the construction of secular or civic monuments. Most monuments and statues exalted the struggles against foreign intervention and domination, and some made explicit reference to Mexico's pre-Hispanic past.

There were also other types of public space — International Exhibitions and archaeological sites. The Great Exhibitions, *Expositions Universelles* or World's Fairs — as they were known in Britain, France and the Unites States respectively — constituted key sites for the display of the progress reached by the nations participating. The industrial, artistic and scientific advances accomplished were lavishly displayed in these international settings, the first of which took place in London in 1851. For the 1889 *Exposition Universelle* held in Paris, doctor and engineer Antonio Peñafiel and engineer Antonio M. Anza designed the *Mexican Pavilion*, and according to Peñafiel the pavilion represented the "purest Aztec style."[30]

The use of Mexico's pre-Hispanic past aimed at legitimizing and consolidating the Porfirian regime both nationally and in the international arena by presenting a unified image of the nation and of its unique origin. A factor that contributed to the appeal of pre-Hispanic *antigüedades* was the increasing interest in the exploration of Mexico's subsoil following the archaeological findings of the time.[31] Simultaneously, the erection of monuments in Mexico City during the Porfiriato led to the use of Mexico's pre-Hispanic past as propaganda.[32] Public space was used as a site for the display of the centralization of economic and political power, and as a site for the display of the state-sponsored official version of history, where the figure of Cuauhtémoc — the last Aztec emperor — asserted the supremacy of the valley and city of Mexico over the rest of the nation.

Monuments and the 1877 Decree

Through the erection of monuments during the last quarter of the nineteenth century, the government attempted to transform the image and appearance of the city in specific places and to legitimize, through the manifestation of its past, its place in national and international history. Although the aesthetic model in the design of monuments was predominately classicism, some incorporated indigenous topics or native decorative elements for the first time. The use of indigenous subjects and/or elements was associated with the idea of the nation, and these elements were regarded as a reaction to foreign intervention and domination, such as the Spanish colonial heritage, the French Intervention (1862–67), and to the new threat posed by the United States, explicitly denounced by Justo Sierra in 1883. Sierra held that Mexico suffered from a triple threat of "Americanism": legal, economic and cultural.[33]

The display in the plastic arts of the men who had fought for the country appealed to a romantic depiction of secular history, and once the Porfiriato secured what was believed to be social peace (after 1884), it claimed to be the successor to the great figures of liberalism. Aesthetic ideas became more utilitarian, in the sense that they linked art with politics and with the plastic representation of the nation. The siting of monuments in public space was very important. Through them, the state usurped the position previously occupied by the Church. This was to some extent the legacy of the Laws of Reform that had separated church and state, and which stressed the victory of liberalism over conservatism, monarchy and foreign intervention. Public monuments were also regarded as educational vehicles or tools that could guide the young and imbue them with moral and civic lessons as well as encourage them to respect and adhere to the laws of the nation.

During the late nineteenth century, the demand for public secular monuments went beyond all bounds throughout Western Europe and the United States, and within this proliferation of monuments Mexico did not lag behind.[34] Monuments — civic monuments — became a key component of the cult of national memory. They aimed to provide historical legitimacy for the Porfirian regime and to support and/or complement the elaboration of an official version of history. Their construction required that they be commissioned by a private or public body due to the financial costs involved, and their siting in a public space required the involvement of the state or local government in the official authorization of the theme, iconography, materials and style. Monuments which honoured the image of a person or a group of persons or an idea (such as Cuauhtémoc, Juárez and Independence) had to be accepted by official representatives. In most cases they were commissioned, supervised and unveiled by the government. Monuments froze a moment in history and constituted a space of triumph and/or of reflection and became a visual homage to memory. They revived past historical events and immobilized important historical figures or moments of history, reinforced the idea that certain dates and names should not be forgotten, and constituted a way of writing history in the urban landscape.

Monuments also served as landmarks or signals, as definers of a specific place, as a focal point for pedestrian and vehicular traffic. The monuments to Independence, Cuauhtémoc, the statues of the Aztec kings Ahuítzotl and Itzcóatl, as well as the thirty-six statues of Mexico's most outstanding men, were sited along the Paseo de la Reforma, an avenue that was regarded an important site. Their placement along this avenue reinforced the symbolic importance of this area of the city and further divided it by making specific areas more valuable (as land prices tended to increase) and prestigious than others.

The Porfirian monuments and statues also shared the use of a set of pre-established aesthetic mandates, that is, the use of historically accepted symbols. Most of these symbols were of classical origin — Greek and Roman — and classicism in monuments and in sculpture gave them universal connotations. For instance, for bravery

> the figure could have its hands clenched and its armed raised as for battle; for justice a standing or sitting lady, blindfolded and holding a pair of scales and a sword, and for beauty, a girl-woman or a boy-man ... Kings, generals and presidents must ride horses, even if they never did ...[35]

The use of large bases added greater stature to the figure by raising it well above eye level, inspiring in the spectators a sense of respect, and making of the monument an inescapable sight. Monuments attempted to make manifest who owned or controlled the power of the visible, but above all, they represented the secular cult of memory and became *"les lieux de mémoire."*[36]

National unity was a paramount concern during the Porfiriato. One of the major objectives of the government was political reconciliation, which meant reconciliation of the factions in conflict within the triumphant liberal party and with the opposition. Among the issues continuously stressed by the government were social peace and economic progress, as well as the final victory of liberalism over conservatism, monarchy and foreign intervention. This climate of political reconciliation was seen as having been made possible by the order and progress of the country brought about by Díaz, and as a direct result of the Reform movement led by Benito Juárez. An important element that helped to shape this discourse of political reconciliation was the attempt to define and promote a sense of national identity, and this was done by searching in history for exemplary actions, events, dates and names. According to Barbara Tenenbaum, there were two main ideological frameworks that guided the erection of specific monuments on public space during the Porfiriato. She names these opposing ideologies the "francophile progressives" and the "nationalist mythologizers" — two distinct groups — formed by conservatives and liberals respectively. Tenenbaum argues that the "francophile progressives" embraced Paris because of its modernity and because they regarded it as the centre of civilization, culture and progress. The "nationalist mythologizers," however, regarded urban renewal and the construction of monuments and buildings as a vehicle for their ideas.[37] The leading representative of the "francophile progressives" was, according to this schema, Antonio Escandón, and the leading "nationalist mythologizer" was General Vicente Riva Palacio, Development Minister during the first presidency of General Porfirio Díaz. In the following pages, reference will be made to both Riva Palacio and Escandón, but instead of attempting to delineate such clear-cut divisions between liberals and conservatives, a task that in itself would constitute the theme for a thorough study, what will be stressed is that Mexico's post-independence chaos was filled with large-scale unifying figures who aimed to inculcate loyalty to the state.

With the following words, the Minister of Development, Vicente Riva Palacio, issued a decree in 1877 that launched a number of artistic competitions for the design of monuments in the capital:

> Public monuments exist not only to perpetuate the memory of heroes and of great men who deserve the gratitude of the people, but also to awaken in some and strengthen in others the love of legitimate glories and also the love of art, where in those monuments one of its most beautiful expressions is to be found. To create recreational areas or boulevards, is to distract members of society with licit diversions within reach of all and allow them to mingle while avoiding the isolation and the vices which are common in populations which lack those means of communication.[38]

Monuments were regarded as constituting visual scenarios with a defined purpose. They were to be visible representations of the men and heroes who had fought for the nation, educational vehicles for both historical and aesthetic sensibility, and erecting them in the city was regarded as conducive to the creation of socially and morally acceptable public areas of communal distraction. The creation of such sites of recreation was important in counteracting the isolation that characterized urban agglomerations, which too often led to vices and illicit means of socialization, issues thoroughly examined by public health officials and hygienists during the Porfiriato.

The 1877 decree was the first deliberate state-sponsored project to promote a comprehensive selection and utilization of Mexico's history. The erection of monuments in the city aimed at making visible the rupture with a past historical time, one dominated by the Church, continuous armed struggles, foreign interventions and political and economic uncertainty. It had to be made clear that this was the beginning of a new epoch, whose foundations were to be found in the 1857 Constitution and which had made possible the triumph of liberalism over conservatism, a struggle led by — among others — General Díaz himself. Monuments would also offer the inhabitants of the city a visual representation of a new political and social order and display the technical advances in the fields of construction and engineering, as well as in the arts. Future generations of Mexicans would become aware of their heroes and of their history, the nation be unified, and the embellishment of the city would additionally help to secure foreign investment. The monuments originally conceived of by Porfirio Díaz were the following:

> The President of the Republic, wishing to embellish the Paseo de la Reforma with monuments worthy of the culture of this city, and whose sights remind of the heroism with which the nation fought against the Conquest in the sixteenth century and for the Independence and the Reform in the present ... has decided ... that a monument to Cuautimotzin and to the other caudillos which distinguished themselves in the defense of the *nation* be made; in the next glorieta, another monument to Hidalgo and to the other heroes of the Independence, and in the following glorieta, one to Juárez and the caudillos of the Reform and of the Second Independence. To begin with this decree ... an artistic competition is opened for the project for the monument destined to Cuautimotzin and the other caudillos who heroically fought against the Conquest.[39]

The site chosen to display the different stages of Mexico's history was the Paseo de la Reforma, the axis of the modern city, along which some of the new *colonias* stood. This area of the city required its own monuments. The central district of the city — the Plaza Mayor — was already symbolically and materially charged. It had been the core of Tenochtitlán; the Spaniards had built the colonial city upon the ruins of the Aztec city, and the Cathedral, the National Palace and the Plaza Mayor had all been witnesses of and participants in the most diverse events throughout the history of the capital city. In contrast, the Paseo was neither symbolically nor materially occupied. Therefore, the modern city would be embellished through the erection of monuments that had as common denominator the struggle of the country against foreign intervention and domination, and would highlight Porfirian peace and order.

As previously mentioned, 1877 was also the year in which a monument to Columbus was unveiled in the second of the *glorietas* of the Paseo de la Reforma, and according to Justino Fernández, it is probable that this monument influenced President Díaz to issue the decree.[40] This monument was a gift to the city from railroad entrepreneur Antonio Escandón, and it was donated to commemorate the opening of his railroad to Veracruz, the Ferrocarril Mexicano, which in 1873 linked Mexico City to the most important commercial port. The French sculptor Charles Henri Joseph Cordier (1827–1905) was commissioned in 1873 to design the statue in Paris, and the statue reached Veracruz in 1875. Two years later, its siting on the Paseo de la Reforma under the supervision of engineer Eleuterio Méndes was finally concluded.[41] And just as Columbus had opened Europe to new possibilities of expansion, wealth and opportunities, the railroad — the symbol of progress of the nineteenth century — had shortened distances, revolutionized the movement of people, goods and capital, and the modern technology used to make them was both highly visible and audible to all.[42] Escandón, imbued with the technological optimism of the age, decided to commemorate the era of the railroad in Mexico with a monument to an equally epochal event, the Discovery of the New World. Thus the monumental endeavour along the Paseo de la Reforma began.

The embellishment of the city and the erection of monuments were also directed towards possible foreign investors, as they endowed the city with an international quality. This internationalism was important because many cities during the late nineteenth century, such as London, Paris, Chicago and St. Louis, Missouri, hosted International Exhibitions or World's Fairs. During those international gatherings, which took place with the purpose of displaying the advances attained in the arts, industry and science, monuments, public buildings and statues were unveiled, and avenues, schools and public works inaugurated which stressed what was being accomplished. Why should Mexico City be excluded from the privilege of hosting one of these prestigious displays of wealth and power? During Riva Palacios' tenure as Minister of Development (1876-1879), the idea of hosting an International Exhibition in the capital with the participation of all the states of the Republic and the most advanced European and American nations led to the creation of a commission devoted to this purpose. The commission included Riva Palacio, Francisco Sosa, Justo Sierra and engineer Francisco Jiménez, among others, and their involvement was such that they even had a weekly publication: *La Exposición Internacional Mexicana*. However, President Díaz disapproved of the proposal because he saw in Riva Palacio a potential presidential candidate and a strong opponent in the 1880 election. Riva Palacio therefore resigned in 1879.[43] The ambition of hosting an International Exhibition in the capital was partially fulfilled during the Centennial Celebrations of Mexico's Independence in 1910.

The Paseo de la Reforma was also selected as the most appropriate site for a tribute that each state of the country was asked to donate to the capital: two life-size bronze statues of their most outstanding men, such as heroes, statesmen, poets, writers, men of science and philanthropists.[44] This request makes evident the symbolic centralization of political and economic power in the capital. The idea of siting statues all along the pavements of the Paseo belonged to Francisco Sosa and was approved by the government on 1 October 1887. Nonetheless, the writer Manuel Gutiérrez Nájera was completely against the tribute paid to the city by the states of the Republic, and exclaimed: "Why should they pay for our festivities? Mexico City is not the Holy Land, it is not a Holy City."[45] However, between 5 February 1889 and 2 April 1899, thirty-six statues were unveiled and inaugurated by government representatives, and it was as "if the rest of the republic was once again paying tribute to its capital as it had done centuries before."[46] Throughout the country, provincial governments followed developments in the capital, and numerous statues were inaugurated in public plazas, important streets and buildings. In the press, the proliferation of statues and monuments was considered a positive element that would educate the people and imbue them with "love for beauty":

> The idea of filling the gardens and public avenues with statues is not just to immortalize great men, but to promote art and to educate the taste of the people, instilling them with a love for beauty. Well it seems that sculptors and architects deploy their talents in the wide field that statue making offers them. Art gains much and history loses nothing.[47]

Cuauhtémoc

According to the 1877 decree, the first monument that had to be erected was one to honour the defence of the nation led by Cuauhtémoc. However, it is important to note that a small monument had previously been made to honour the last Aztec Emperor. In 1869, the base supporting a small grey bust of the last Aztec Emperor — sculpted by Manuel Islas — was placed in the Paseo de la Viga. The inauguration of this tribute was more impressive than the monument itself. President Juárez, his cabinet, Mexico City's governor and the entire Municipal Council were present for the solemn occasion.[48] By contrast, in 1877 it was clearly specified that the monument was to be erected in the most prestigious avenue of the city, and its dimensions, cost and publicity far exceeded the 1869 small grey bust. Five designs were submitted in 1877 to a committee led by Vicente Riva Palacio that included the English graphic artist Juan Santiago Baggally and architects Emilio Dondé Preciat, Ramón Rodríguez Arangoity and Manuel Gargollo y Parra. The project that won the competition belonged to Francisco Jiménez and had as its theme *Verdad, Belleza y Utilidad*, referring to historical truth, artistic beauty and moral utility.[49] Jiménez thought that the most appropriate architectural and stylistic characteristics of his project relied on borrowing details from the ruins of Tula, Uxmal, Mitla and Palenque, and on "conserving as much as possible the general character of the architecture of the ancient inhabitants of this Continent." This would allow him to create a "characteristic style," a "national style."[50] The emphasis on creating a national style by incorporating details of non-Aztec cultures and from the most diverse regions of the country to represent Cuauhtémoc, the defender of Tenochtitlán — Mexico City — indicate the centralization of political power taking place at the time and the appropriation of other indigenous cultures by the capital.

It is important to note that the use of the figure of the Indian and of pre-Hispanic cultures in painting and sculpture throughout the course of the nineteenth century was inextricably linked to the liberal revolution, which involved a gradual replacement of religious iconography with patriotic exaltation in the arts. The first time in independent Mexico that an indigenous theme was represented in sculpture was in 1850, when the artist Manuel Vilar (1812–60, Barcelona), who arrived in Mexico in

1846 to head the sculpture department of the Academia de San Carlos, produced a sculpture of Moctezuma II. The display of Moctezuma II represented the advent in Mexico of the use of pre-Hispanic motives and themes in "high-art."[51] In painting, during the second half of the nineteenth century, and in particular after 1867, a number of large historical works also portrayed events from the pre-Hispanic past. According to Ida Rodríguez,[52] the figure of the Indian first appeared in 1850, when, kneeling down or in a submissive attitude, he entered the Academy in Juan Cordero's *Colón ante los Reyes Católicos*.[53] Forty-five years later, on the morning of 21 October 1895, the newspaper *El Siglo XIX* gave an account of a tour that the delegates of the Congress of Americanists made in the Academia de Bellas Artes to view some paintings that, after four centuries of artistic production, depicted the figure of the Mexican Indian. They were particularly impressed with the following: *El tormento de Cuauhtémoc* by Leandro Izaguirre; *La prisión de Cuauhtémoc*, by Joaquín Ramírez; *Visita de Cortés a Moctezuma*, by Juan Ortega; *El Senado de Tlaxcala*, by Rodrigo Gutiérrez; *Fray Bartolomé de las Casas protector de Indios* by Félix Parra; *La reina Xóchitl ofreciendo el pulque al rey azteca,* by José Obregón; and *Episodios de la conquista*, by Félix Parra, among others.[54]

The handful of paintings that had as their theme the Indian and the pre-Hispanic past appeared clothed in neo-classical style, and were of a magnitude that recalls the paintings done by Jacques-Louis David (1748–1825) to commemorate the French Revolution, whose themes gave expression to the new cult of the civic virtues of stoical self-sacrifice, devotion to duty, honesty and austerity. However, while David was inspired by the Roman emperors and by the classical past, Mexican artists looked to their native past for scenes and motives to depict. In monuments, only Cuauhtémoc — the last Aztec emperor, as he was generally referred to — and two monumental statues of Ahuítzotl and Itzcóatl by the sculptor Alejandro Casarín, paid homage to the city the Aztecs had once dominated.

The first stone of Cuauhtémoc's monument was laid on 5 May 1878, one of the key dates in Mexico's civic calendar. After Jiménez's death in 1884, the project was continued by architect and engineer Ramón Agea. Miguel Noreña was responsible for sculpting the figure of Cuauhtémoc, the base of the monument and one of the bas-reliefs representing the *Prisión de Cuauhtémoc*. Sculptors Jesús F. Contreras and Gabriel Guerra also collaborated. The monument was inaugurated on 21 August 1887, cost some 97,914 pesos, weighed 11,908 kilograms in bronze, and numerous reviews, studies, poems and celebrations surrounded the civic event.[55]

What is important to stress is the reappraisal and utilization of Mexico's pre-Hispanic past, and in particular the notion that Cuauhtémoc's courage, stoicism and patriotism, constituted characteristics that the Mexican people could acquire if properly taught, reflecting the confidence the proponents of triumphant liberalism had in education. The other aspect I wish to stress is that the technological progress that made possible the construction of the monument was also visible and tangible evidence of the technological progress of the nation.

On 21 August 1887, General Porfirio Díaz, military and civil authorities, students and representatives of different indigenous communities were present at the inauguration. An official address was made by Alfredo Chavero, the National Anthem was played by a military band, poetry was read out and a speech in Nahuatl was given by Francisco del Paso y Troncoso. The program of activities set out for the day was published in most newspapers of the capital, such as the *Diario del Hogar*.[56] The unveiling of this monument, as well as that of all others, was a civic ceremony, a cultural depiction of how things should be. Through it, the state aimed to display public order, hierarchy, a common social identity as well as public consensus. The ceremony can also be interpreted as a public dramatization of the city's ability of represent itself. As all the guests and the public proceeded to their destination, to the established civic centre, they professed loyalty to their leader, to the values, beliefs and aspirations of the government. The state, through this monument, aimed at portraying a much sought-after national unity.

Cuauhtémoc — the hero of resistance — is represented in a military role, as if prepared for battle: his right arm is raised holding a spear, his face is calm and determined, and his body is supported in the classical manner of *contraposto*. His right leg is set back, and the weight rests on his left foot, making the figure appear to advance when viewed from the side, yet to be stationary when viewed from the front. According to Marina Warner, the incorporation of any specific historical reference can endanger an image's survival as a symbol. Therefore, it was decided to rely on classical representations of specific allegories to give the work universal connotations.[57] For Carlos Monsiváis,

Cuauhtémoc's monument represents the beginning of a reconciliation with the past: "At long last, there was an Indian hero to represent — not ethnic pride (unthinkable in Díaz's time) — but rather, the beginning of a reconciliation with the past. He was an Indian, but he was an emperor."[58] Cuauhtémoc's monument honoured a mythical ancient past (see Figure 2).

Ahuítzotl and Itzcóatl

Two less popular bronze statues, representing the Aztec kings Itzcóatl and Ahuítzotl, were inaugurated on 16 September 1891.[59] Each statue was 5.9 metres in height, with a weight of more than four tons, and their pedestals were made of black national marble by the sculptor Alejandro Casarín. Originally the statues were made for display at the 1889 *Exposition Universelle* in Paris, but instead they were erected on the Paseo de la Reforma. After their inauguration, they were referred to by the inhabitants of the city as 'Indios Verdes' and became the object of criticism and satire in the press:

> At the entrance to the Paseo ... there are two colossal green oxidized bronze statues. I send you the photo of the characters for you to see ... these figures are occupying a place which by law corresponds to them in the national foundry. What beautiful cannons would come out of them! Imagine that looking at them from afar, from very far away, they look like fetuses outside a bottle.[60]

In 1900, when the city was repeatedly being praised for its buildings and for its cosmopolitan character, and when an increasing number of reviews made public the archaeological findings within the city following the excavations carried out during the installation of sewers and drinking water, a guide to the city made the following remarks about the two Aztec kings:

> The first thing that one sees at the beginning of the Paseo is a pair of monsters, that is to say a pair of colossi Aztecs cast in bronze and which are two monsters engendered in the mind of someone who does not have the slightest idea of aesthetics.[61]

The criticisms of the Indios Verdes continued, and *El Imparcial* was very happy to inform its readers that a solution was soon to be given: they were to be removed from the Paseo. In their

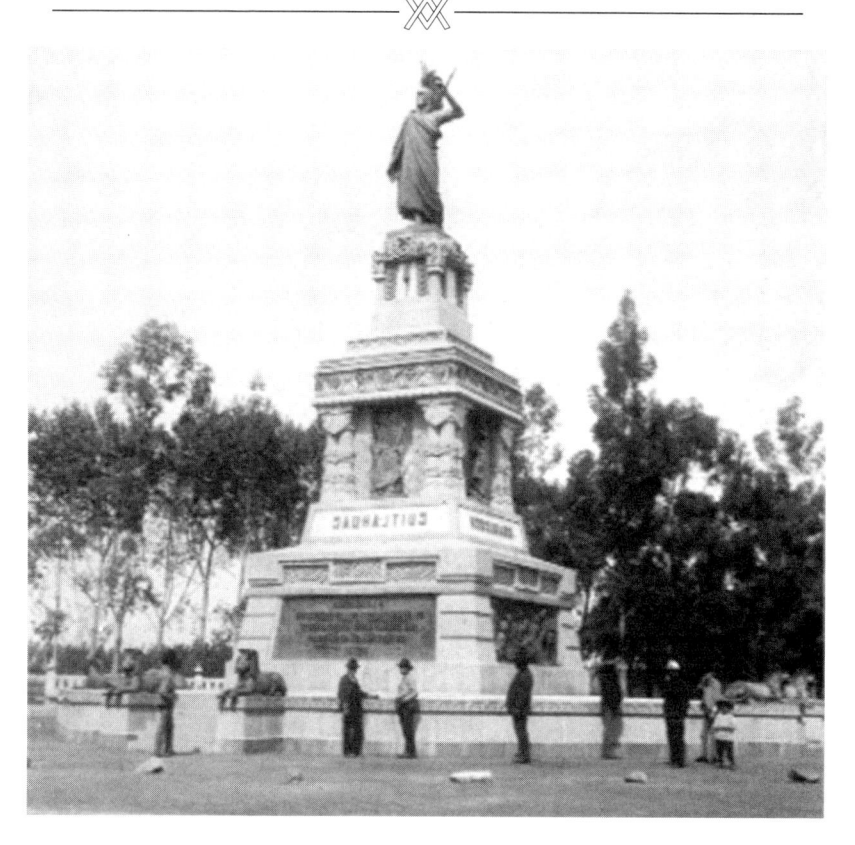

Figure 2. Monument to Cuauhtémoc, 1901.
© CONACULTA-INAH-SINAFO-FOTOTECA NACIONAL DEL INAH, Mexico.

place, two artistic pillars, following the model of those that stood on the Piazza of St. Marcos, in Venice, would be placed at the entrance to the Paseo de la Reforma.[62] In 1901, the Indios Verdes were moved to the old unsanitary city, to the Paseo de la Viga, and stood near the site of the first monument to honour Cuauhtémoc (see Figure 3). By 1904, this area of the city housed many factories and was well known for its litter, open ditches and sewers. The stench emanating from its stagnant water was additionally aggravated by an unacceptable practice: the use of the open ditches as toilets by the urban population.[63] This area of the city was deliberately excluded from the imagery of modernity.

In the modern city, the view of its inhabitants was no longer obstructed by the figures of the two Aztec kings who were not

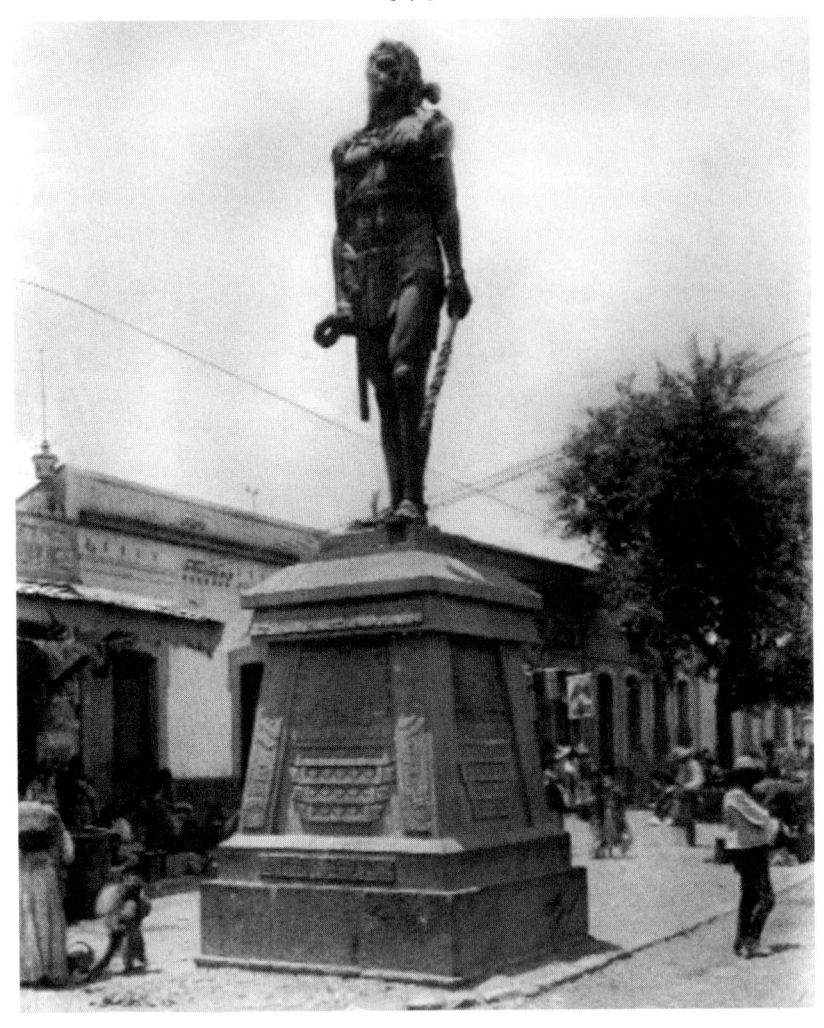

Figure 3. Indio Verde on the Calzada de la Viga, 1907.
© CONACULTA-INAH-SINAFO-FOTOTECA NACIONAL DEL INAH, MEXICO.

as fortunate as Cuauhtémoc. However, a few remaining visible ancient monuments had still to be demolished: the aqueducts. Aqueducts were seen not only as aesthetically dull and as an obstacle to the lengthening of the streets, but also as potential threats to public health.[64] Water, it was argued, had to reach all homes and buildings by a system of underground pipes, and in 1882 it was agreed that the Arcos de Belem had to be taken down because they were an obstruction to the widening of the streets and to the visual impact of the modern city.[65] In 1896, it was argued that the arches of the aqueduct that surrounded the Bosque de Chapultepec should go. The stones would be used for the embellishment of the park, and for paving some city streets.[66] In 1900, some arches of the Chapultepec aqueduct still remained because they had been classified as 'ancient monuments,' but it was nevertheless held that they hindered the visual aspect of the avenue upon which they stood.[67] Architect Leopoldo Salazar wrote to the Municipal Council on 5 December 1900 demanding that no more arches be demolished, but the response he received stated that there was no good reason to preserve those primitive and ugly arches.[68]

As aqueducts were being demolished, streets enlarged and paved and artistic competitions held for the construction of monuments, buildings and statues, concern regarding the visual character of the city was growing. By 1900, the city had expanded considerably, and the Municipal Council had been unable to provide basic urban infrastructure for the numerous new housing areas, in spite of the fact that in that same year the drainage works were inaugurated. Particularly worrying was the lack of sanitary installations, both private and public. In 1904, the Superior Sanitation Council urged the Municipal Council not to allow new buildings within the city unless they had adequate sanitary facilities for the workers.[69] Not only were the numerous builders employed in the construction sites seen as possible threats to public health due to the lack of sanitary facilities, but the factories within the city, and even those that cast metal for the new statues and monuments, were denounced by the inhabitants of the affected areas. In 1905, the inhabitants of the *colonia* Juárez expressed their anger and concern in a letter to the Municipal Council, and demanded a prompt solution. They argued that the industrial establishment was hazardous to their health, that the smoke and dust damaged their properties and that the continuous noise was unbearable.[70] Those demands made explicit reference to the Sanitary Code issued in 1891. Chapter 5 of the Sanitary Code (articles 120–200; in particular articles 120, 121, 130–32, 137 and 138) clearly set down that any industrial establishment classified as hazardous to public health had to be located far away from populated areas, in the outskirts or suburbs of the city.[71] But the fact was that the Sanitary Code was seldom respected or enforced.

Benito Juárez and Independence

According to the 1877 decree, a monument to the Reform and to the Second Independence (the Restored Republic of 1867–76 was referred to as the "Second Independence") also had to be erected, and what is important to stress at this point is that it was during the Porfiriato that the glorification of the leader of the Reform and of the "Second Independence," Benito Juárez, began. The official manipulation of a Juárez myth was carried out through celebrations, eulogistic studies, textbooks and poetry, as well as through literary and historical essays and competitions. The purpose was to establish a continuity between Díaz's policies and those of Juárez, even though the two leaders had been enemies.[72] The aim was to "invent a tradition."[73] By appealing to Juárez's legacy of reform, democracy, independence and self-determination, the Díaz regime aimed to anchor itself in the recent past, and with this purpose in mind established the fifteenth anniversary of Juárez's death — 18 July 1887 — as a major national festival. In the midst of the celebrations, a pamphlet written by Marcial Aznar was published, and in it the author argued that Juárez was the symbol of the race and of the nation, as he had saved democracy and reinforced the system of popular representation. Juárez had placed Mexico on an equal footing with European nations and had issued the Laws of Reform to combat ecclesiastical errors. Not only that, Aznar added, but before Juárez, Mexico had been the plaything of European powers.[74] By selectively exalting Juárez's accomplishments, history was used to legitimize Díaz's policies and establish a foundation of his government.

During the 1890s, a national commission for the construction of a monument to Juárez was set up. It was made up of distinguished and wealthy members of the Porfirian elite who argued that Juárez's monument should portray republicanism, liberty and justice.[75] These values became embodied in the figure of the Indian Juárez. His monument was originally planned to occupy one roundabout along the Paseo de la Reforma, but siting it on the most prestigious avenue of the city might overshadow the figure of Porfirio Díaz. Therefore, it was decided that the most appropriate site was next to the Alameda, in the avenue that bears Benito Juárez's name.

The project that won the competition belonged to architect Guillermo de Heredia and was designed as follows: in the centre of a semicircle of twelve doric columns made of white Carrara marble stands the central pedestal supporting the statues of three figures. One statue represents former president Juárez,

> who appears solemn and grim as a Roman proconsul administering justice. Juárez the law-giver is seated, and surrounding him are two female allegories. One is a winged female representing Victory and Glory, who is placing a garland of Victory on Juárez's head. The other figure represents Justice, who stands behind, resting her sword on the ground to signify the end of a gigantic struggle. Crowned by a doric frieze, the columns support a massive, ornate bronze urn at each end, and at the foot of the central pedestal, decorated in gold-plated figures and letters, below the national eagle, rest two marble lions.[76]

The entire monument weighed 1,625 tons and occupied 510 square metres. Juárez's statue alone weighed seventy tons, was seven metres high and was fashioned by the Italian sculptor Lazaroni. The total cost of the monument was 390,065.98 pesos, and it was completed in only ten months.[77] When this massive monument was inaugurated on 18 September 1910, during the centennial celebrations of Mexico's Independence, the following comment was made:

> The Republic would have failed in one of its duties, if in this celebrations it had neglected to honor in a significant manner, the grand figure of the patriot and statesmen whose entire life was dedicated to ensuring the reign of justice and law, as the political base that inspired his solid and far-seeing judgement, maintained and applied tenaciously through his love of the fatherland.[78]

However, by being placed in a semicircle of white marble and classical composition, Juárez was deprived of his Indian roots: "Juárez, we have raised to you statues modeled not with blood and human ashes, like the Aztec semi-gods, but with marbles and bronzes as indestructible as your own work," as Carlos Robles expressed.[79] By stripping away Juárez's identity and likening his achievements to those of ancient Western lawgivers and heroes, Díaz could then praise and use him to legitimize his own long domination of the country. What the Díaz regime wished to exalt was the political legacy of the Reform, the Constitution of 1857, and the final defeat over foreign intervention and conservative ideology, and Juárez and many of his liberal colleagues became synonymous with Mexican nationalism (see Figure 4).[80]

Through this monument, the Díaz regime wished to represent the foundation of his government, and identified its struggles with those led by Juárez between 1858 and 1872. It aimed to conceal the differences between Juárez's and Díaz's achievements, and to exalt the figure not of a mythical Indian like Cuauhtémoc but of an Indian who had become president and who had responded to the contemporary universal values of republicanism, liberty and justice:[81] "Did not Juárez ascend from being a simple shepherd from the hills of Ixtlán to the supreme dignities of the Republic?"[82]

The other key monument for the city was that erected to the Independence of Mexico. In 1901, the project was commissioned to Antonio Rivas Mercado (1853–1926), a French-trained architect who had lived in Paris and London and who was a keen follower of the Paris Beaux Arts style.[83] The requirements set out by the government regarding the monument specified that it had to be a commemorative column and that it was to be placed in the fourth *glorieta* of the Paseo de la Reforma, which had a diameter of two hundred metres. Rivas Mercado's project bore some resemblance to the commemorative column conceived during the presidency of Antonio López de Santa Anna by Lorenzo de la Hidalga on 23 August 1843, a project that was taken up again by Emperor Maximilian in 1865. On all three occasions (1843, 1865 and 1901), the aim was to build a commemorative column with a group of allegorical sitting figures, above which would stand a winged victory, the quintessential representation of republican liberty throughout the nineteenth century.[84] Neither Hidalga's nor Maximilian's project was executed, due to political instability and the financial costs involved, but on those occasions it was thought that the most suitable site for the column was at the centre of the Plaza Mayor. By 1901, the chosen site was no longer the Plaza Mayor. The Paseo de la Reforma was selected instead, regardless of the fact that opposition mounted when this idea was confirmed, as expressed by Jesús Galindo y Villa, among others.[85]

The construction began in 1902, and architect Rivas Mercado was responsible for the entire project and its artistic style. The Italian sculptor Enrique Alciati made all the statues and the ornamentation. The works continued without interruption until

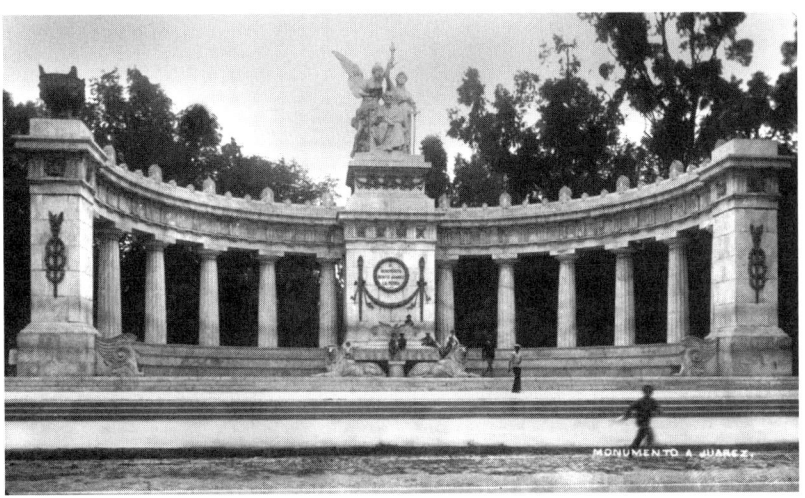

Figure 4. Monument to Benito Juárez, 1911.
© CONACULTA-INAH-SINAFO-FOTOTECA NACIONAL DEL INAH, Mexico.

1906, when they had to be suspended because the foundations were not strong enough to support the base or the weight of the column. To solve the technical problems, a commission to undertake all the engineering work was formed by engineers Guillermo Beltrán y Puga, Gonzalo Garitas and Manuel Marroquín y Rivera. When it was finally inaugurated in 1910, the column, 45.16 metres in height, on top of which rests the figure of a golden winged angel, became the highest and most visible landmark of the capital, as well as the most expensive. Its total cost amounted to approximately 2,146,704 pesos.[86]

The monument consists of a terrace upon which the base of the column rests. The base has a bronze statue of a lion and a small boy representing a genius; "the lion, laden with laurels and guided by a genius, represents the Mexican people who cover themselves with the laurels and who are submissive and obedient to duty."[87] Each corner has four bronze figures, representing Peace, Law, Justice and War. The names of twenty-four men who fought for Independence are also engraved. The base of the monument has a door that leads to a number of crypts and to the stairs that lead to the top of the column. On the next level of the base, where the column properly begins, stands the marble figure of Hidalgo facing the city. He is surrounded by the marble figures of Morelos, Guerrero, Mina and Nicolás

Bravo, one in each corner. All the marble statues were made in Carrara, Italy, by sculptor Enrique Alciati; the bronze statues were made in Florence and the decorations in Paris. At Hidalgo's feet are two female figures, one representing History and the other the Motherland. At the top of the column stands the huge figure of a golden angel. The symbol of Victory and Independence is 6.7 metres tall and weighs seven thousand kilograms. In its left hand it holds a fragment of a chain, and in its right a crown.[88] In 1910, a study of this monument established that it had a majestic design, but that is was also simple and sincere. Above all, it had the virtue of not belonging to any given historical period or aesthetic mandate. Thus, it was classical but also modern, as well as neo-classical.[89] It fixed history, in particular Mexico's Independence, in no specific time or moment and placed it above time and place, just as some religious symbols tend to represent timelessness through their presence. The winged angel, which symbolizes success, glory, fame and victory, is a metaphor for time's halt, which is implicit in the figure of the Greek goddess of Victory, and this freezing of time was the intention of this monument. Its height made it an unavoidable sight, and it could be viewed from most areas of the city. The origin of the extended and embracing wings of victory was in heaven, in the world above:[90] "The column rises up to the firmament like the eternal aspiration of man toward superior forms of life... above the capital ... an angel opens its wings in whom we confuse 'Independence' and 'Victory!'"[91] (see Figure 5).

The erection of monuments in the city by the Porfirian regime aimed to display the different stages of Mexican history for all to see, as well as to underline and reinforce the ideas of "nation," "progress" and "peace." Thus, the modern city held within it the pre-Hispanic past (Cuauhtémoc, Itzcóatl and Ahuítzotl), the Discovery of America (Columbus), the colonial period (the statue of Charles IV), the Second Independence (Juárez's monument) and Mexico's Independence, as well as the most prominent men and heroes of Mexico's historical, artistic, literary and scientific heritage. Through the construction of monuments, but even more so during the unveiling rituals that accompanied the inauguration of statues, monuments and busts, the Porfirian elite presented an image of itself and of its place in history. The processions to the monumental sites, the hierarchy of those present, the speeches and poetry read by prominent politicians and men of letters, as well as the historical reconstruction performed for each occasion, all underlined the impression that the Porfirian regime had made possible Mexico's modernization. The Porfiriato was the culmination of Mexico's historical development; it was the pinnacle of the political evolution of the Mexican nation. Justo Sierra defined the Porfiriato in his essay *La evolución política del pueblo Mexicano* as an era of peace during which the Mexican nation had acquired its international personality.[92] Mexico's peace, order, progress and internationalism were emphasized during the inaugurations for each monument. And monuments, like murals later on, entrusted the nation's heroes with a mission, that of stressing the successful and harmonious continuity of the system.[93]

When the monument to Independence was inaugurated, at ten in the morning of 16 September 1910, the President was accompanied by all the members of his government, by the numerous foreign guests who had been invited to Mexico's Centennial Celebrations (or to its own *Exposition Universelle*), as well as by the army and the police. The National Anthem was played, the National Flag and National Emblem displayed, and the poem *Al Buen Cura* was read by Salvador Díaz Mirón.[94] Official speeches were made by leading members of Mexico City's Municipal Council and of the Ministry of the Interior. Miguel Macedo's speech emphasized that the Independence

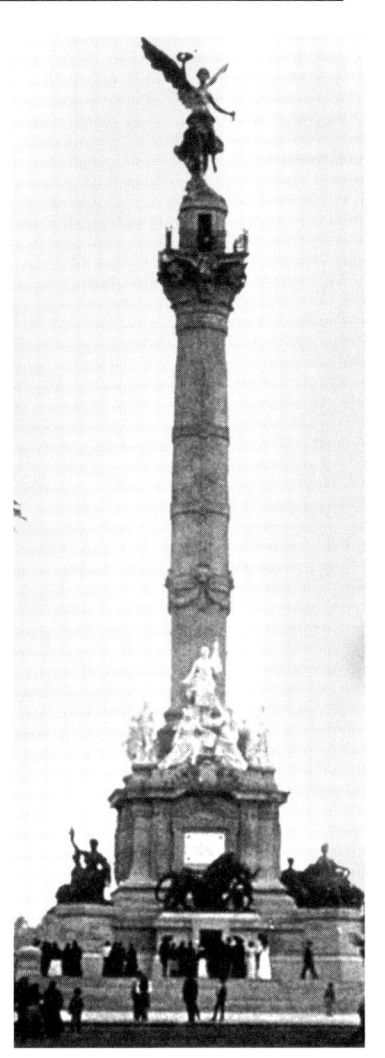

Figure 5. Monument to Independence.
Source: Archivo Fotográfico Instituto de Investigaciones Estéticas – UNAM, Mexico City. Reproduction authorized by the Instituto Nacional de Bellas Artes y Literatura, Mexico (Photograph by L.B. García).

movement that had begun in 1810 without organization or discipline had led to an entire century of unending work towards independence, and that the era of order, peace and progress had made possible the construction of the monument.[95]

Monumental Space and Cleanliness

Endowing the city with monuments worthy of any other major city of the world was important in displaying Mexico's order, progress and technical and scientific achievements. However, monumental space had to be clean. In the previous chapters, I have shown that the goal of hygienists, the Municipal Council and the Superior Sanitation Council was to attain a hygienic, ordered and clean city. The worries about the possibility of contagion and disease led to a war on dirt, and this intensified during the years preceding the inauguration of Juárez's monument and the Column of Independence, in the midst of the celebrations of Mexico's Independence in 1910.[96] Three years before the Centennial Celebrations, the Superior Sanitation Council requested that all sanitary inspectors make detailed reports of the conditions found in all public sanitary kiosks (public watercloakers) throughout the city. The result of the inquiry was submitted to the Superior Sanitation Council on 8 February 1908, and their findings were disappointing. Eighteen sanitary kiosks were found scattered throughout the eight quarters of the city in small plazas and public gardens, in sites where large numbers of people often gathered. Conditions in all of them were described as unacceptable, and in one of them were particularly appalling. In the Eighth Quarter of the city, next to the monument to Cuauhtémoc, this sanitary kiosk was described with the following words:

> It is in a very bad state because the top of one of the toilets needs repairing and in another toilet the wooden cover for the bowl is missing; a water installation that works as it should is also needed, because the water tank is not working. Furthermore, one of the urinals does not have a water stopper; the pump intended to feed the water tank which is used to clean the toilets and urinals is broken, the toilets lack a ventilation tube and part of the tiles of the walls and floors is damaged and finally there is no washbasin, nor towels or paper. [97]

On 20 February 1908, Guillermo B. Puga, General Director of Public Works of the Federal District, informed the owner of the sanitary kiosks, Mr. Vicente Almada, that within thirty days the unsanitary conditions found in all public bathrooms had to be brought into line with the standards established by the Superior Sanitation Council. Almada was told that he had to repair their technical faults and provide them with wash basins, towels and paper. On 16 March 1908, Almada replied and argued that it was useless and unnecessary to supply them with wash basins, towels and paper because ninety per cent of the people who approached those public facilities did so with the aim of stealing all that could be removed, and that anyone wishing to check this could do so by simply reading through the reports at the police stations.[98] The lack of morality of the urban population, he said, was appalling, and the users of those facilities defecated anywhere inside the kiosk, in particular in the urinals, which were free of charge, in order to avoid paying five cents, the cost for using the toilet. Some people, he added, had also been caught having sexual intercourse inside the kiosks.[99] The owners or concession-holders of public bathrooms in tenement buildings and/or public markets did not provide any of the comforts he was required to supply, and not a single theatre or governmental building had them. After his angry outburst he agreed to improve them, arguing that the first sanitary kiosk to be repaired and cleansed would be the one close to Cuauhtémoc's monument.[100]

The Superior Sanitation Council was not alone in being extremely vigilant over the unsanitary conditions in the city. Some sectors of the urban population also expressed their concern and demanded that the city be thoroughly cleansed. For instance, in 1908, a group of neighbours whose homes were close to a new avenue named Cuauhtémotzin — to the south of the Plaza Mayor in the central district of the city — wrote a letter to the Superior Sanitation Council demanding that an open ditch that ran parallel to the avenue be cleansed as soon as possible because it constituted a constant threat to the vicinity and to public health.[101] However, that was not the only motive that moved them to express their discontent:

> At the entrance to this ditch, run the trains which go to the picturesque towns of Tlalpan, Churubusco and Coyoacán, and

> the passengers traveling in them (among them all too frequently foreigners who come to Mexico ...) have to form a very sad idea of the capital on seeing that filthy ditch, and the bad impression they experience is palpable, as it suffices to watch their gestures of displeasure by what they see and the disgusting atmosphere they breathe. The existence of such a ditch, is very repugnant, given that it is a five minute walk from the main square. This part of the city does not progress, yet it should occupy a position of preference given its proximity to the center ...[102]

It was deemed imperative to clean the city in order to suppress the threats to public health, but also to improve the image that visitors, in particular foreign visitors, would have of the capital city. By August 1910, the attempts to cleanse the city were intensified due to the Centennial Celebrations that were to begin the following month. On 13 August, a motion was presented to the Municipal Council by Leopoldo Flores in which he argued that it was essential to clean the capital, to paint the exterior walls of many buildings, to pave streets and to drain and cover all open ditches, especially those close to the *colonias* Maza and Valle-Gómez, areas that made a terrible impression on all visitors who had to cross them in order to reach the central district.

> ... given the *fiestas* with which the first anniversary of the proclamation of Mexican Independence will be celebrated in the capital, this town council has been working so that the city should be as clean as possible for then and that it should give a pleasing appearance to the numerous people who should come to the *fiestas* and undoubtedly many people will take this opportunity to visit the city ... The ditches and litter create a very disagreeable impression on the people ... who come to the city, whether by street car, by carriage or even by foot ...[103]

The governor of the Federal District responded on 29 August, arguing that in spite of the fact that the cleansing of the city was the chief responsibility of the Dirección General de Obras Públicas, the government had ordered the inhabitants of unsanitary areas to clean all streets and open ditches, and giving reassurances that the police would be present to supervise the implementation of these instructions.[104] When the Centennial Celebrations began, it was agreed that during the inauguration of the Monument to Independence, all those attending the ceremony should be clean and properly dressed, wear shoes and behave in an orderly manner. Thus, because it was impossible to keep the urban poor and the indigenous population out of the "modern" city, it was necessary to "camouflage them."[105] However, the most elaborate display of the hygienic, clean, safe and modern city was exhibited during the Popular Hygiene Exhibition (Exposición Popular de Higiene), which opened on 2 September. Here, large numbers of people of all social classes, and in particular the poor, got the opportunity to examine models and furniture and to receive hygienic education, essential requirements for progress and survival.[106]

The deliberate attempt to transform the image of the city during the Porfiriato led to an unprecedented construction fever. For the first time since Independence, the government was able to set aside a substantial amount of resources for the embellishment of the capital and for the construction of public works. Numerous photographs and descriptions of the city continually stressed the lengthening of the streets and the unobstructed views of the city, as well as its buildings and monuments. These material elements stressed the prosperity of the country and the advances accomplished in the fields of construction and engineering, as well as the supremacy of the capital over the rest of the country.

The transformation of the capital was concentrated in specific areas, and its benefits were enjoyed only by a minority of the urban population. While monuments and buildings were inaugurated by General Díaz and members of his cabinet, large sectors of the capital's population were living without any of the advantages that modern technology had brought to the city, and it is more than probable that large sectors of the urban population did not recognize the figures portrayed by the monuments, let alone understand the speech read out in Nahuatl during the inauguration of the statue of Cuauhtémoc.

It must be noted that not everyone praised the government's attempts to embellish the city. In the national press, it was common for journalists to write articles criticizing the public works carried out by the government, claiming that it was more concerned with embellishing the city than with building efficient public works to prevent the chaos that occurred every time it rained. Not only were criticisms levelled by Mexicans; foreigners voiced similar opinions. The North American Charles Flandrau travelled throughout Mexico between 1904 and 1907 and wrote the book *Viva México!* (first published in 1908), in which he gave an account of his first impressions after arriving in the capital.[107] Some of the features he mentioned — asphalted streets, movement of people and cars, noises and lights of a metropolis — could indeed be perceived in certain areas of the city. However, when he wrote that after forty-eight hours the "glitter became increasingly difficult to discern," he reflected the fact that that glitter and metropolitan atmosphere was confined to a specific area of the city, and that those features were nonexistent for large sectors of the urban population. The image of the modern city had numerous flaws. While some sectors of the population identified the modernity of the city with the visual impact some areas were acquiring following the construction of buildings, homes and monuments, there were other visual elements present in the city that could not be part of that modernity, such as the remaining ancient monuments, the aqueducts.

Another factor that shattered the order, hierarchy and aspirations of the Porfirian elite was the behaviour, customs and lack of education of large sectors of the urban population, as well as their lack of cleanliness. Because the cleanliness factor was extremely important, a key problem had to be addressed: the chaos that took over the city due to the lack of an adequate drainage system. Some areas of the city, in particular those close to Lake Texcoco, were still suffering in 1910 from the perennial problems caused by floods, making the circulation of people and goods almost impossible, damaging buildings and homes and impinging directly on the health of the population. It was not enough to have large modern buildings that would be equally at home in Paris or London, or impressive monuments praising the heroes of Mexico's history. It was necessary to clean the city, and to this end, which had already been the focus of effort and thought of generations of Mexicans, the Porfirio Díaz government took on the historic task of making the city safe, clean and modern. This meant completing a monumental public work: the drainage system for the valley and city of Mexico.

5

The Conquest of Water

By the late nineteenth century, the consensus of opinion among public health experts, engineers and the government was that the unsanitary conditions of the capital and its high incidence of premature death and disease would finally be controlled when efficient drainage and sewer systems were built. But their construction was also important on a symbolic level, as they would manifest the monumental achievements of the Porfiriato. The dangers posed by floods and by the overflow of the city's sewers and open ditches was the kind of natural disaster that could be controlled, unlike earthquakes or volcanic eruptions, and the taming of nature became an essential component of the late –nineteenth century idea of progress. The technological and scientific knowledge that made this conquest possible gradually penetrated homes and workplaces, transformed daily lives as well as bodily pleasures, and led to the construction of a vast socio-sanitary domain that altered the landscape both above and below ground.[1]

During the late nineteenth century, it was believed that it was just as important for a city to have an adequate supply of pure water per inhabitant (its purity was, of course, scientifically established) as it was to rid the entrails of the city — the sewers — of waste. In Mexico City, the draining and cleansing of the menacing environment, and thus the conquest of the water that had besieged it throughout its history, was seen as an essential requirement for its prosperity and modernity, and this conquest was also regarded as an indicator of progress and civilization. For instance, in the United States, a Baltimore engineer drew a parallel in 1905 between the efficiency of the sewers and the quality of civilization and, referring to France, argued that "completely sewered, with a low death rate Paris is the center of all that is best in art, literature, science and architecture, and is both clean and beautiful [and] its sewers took at least a leading part."[2] The French sanitary engineer A. Mille argued during the late nineteenth century that the progress in hygiene was to be a revolution perhaps as great as that of the railways, and referred to the new Parisian sewers as the "cloaca maxima," establishing an imperial analogy between the *cloaca maxima* of Ancient Rome and the sewers made possible by modern science and technology.[3] In Mexico City, the progress in public health and the image of the modern capital during the late nineteenth century had much to do with control of the menacing environment, and engineering was regarded as a profession that had the task of fulfilling a key social role: the material and social improvement of the nation. In addition, engineers became the "physicians" of the city and were held to be agents of civilization.[4]

Within this self-appointed civilizing mission of working towards the progress of the nation, the idea that only when water was entirely tamed through the construction of a monumental public work would the city stand on an equal footing with other major cities of the world took hold of the profession, and it was during the Porfiriato that the conquest of water was partially accomplished. The previous pages have shown that disease and epidemics had inspired municipal authorities to install town planning and cleansing measures since the late colonial period, and that in 1891 the Ministry of the Interior issued a Sanitary Code. In addition, the topographical surveys or diagnoses of the city had led public health officials to establish that the lack of sanitation and the inadequate or non-existent hygienic practices of the urban population were an obstacle to progress. Thus, throughout the course of the nineteenth century numerous laws, regulations and measures were implemented in an attempt to keep the city and its inhabitants clean and diminish the impact of disease and epidemics. However, a major factor in keeping the city clean, ordered and hygienic was the control of the flow of tainted water within it.

The Problem:
Water

Since pre-Hispanic times the city had suffered from the impact of floods caused by the overflow of the lakes that surrounded it, and by the overflow of the canals that criss-crossed it. Floods continued throughout the colonial years and during the nineteenth century, and even today, when rainfall is persistent enough, many areas of the city become flooded. During the colonial era, the capital of New Spain was seriously flooded in 1555, 1580, 1604 and 1607. Until 1607, the method of dealing with floods had been the same as that applied by the Aztecs: the building of dikes and dams to protect the city.[5] However, the 1607 flood led to such destruction that Viceroy Luis de Velasco Segundo (Viceroy of New Spain from 1590 to 1595 and from 1607 to 1611) decided that the solution should not rely on containing water but on expelling it from the city and the valley of Mexico. The method conceived was a drainage system. Thus, 1607 is the year when the plan to expel water from the city was first carried out, although it was originally conceived during the mid-sixteenth century.[6] The plan was revived and abandoned throughout the years from 1607 until the late nineteenth century. In 1607, the project involved building a drainage canal, half tunnel and half open trench, which was to guide the floodwaters of the Valley of Mexico through the surrounding mountains of Nochostingo to the northwest of the city into the Tula River, from which they would flow to the Gulf of Mexico.[7] The purpose of the open trench or canal (with a length of six kilometres) was to connect Lake Zumpango to the town of Huehuetoca by cutting across the mountains of Nochostingo. At the end of the canal, a tunnel 6.5 kilometres long would channel into its course all the water from the river Cuautitlán. This tunnel would also help to drain Lake San Cristóbal, prevent the back flow of Lake Texcoco and lower the water level of Lake Mexico. Finally, at the end of the tunnel an open trench 650 metres in length would guide all the water into the river Tula and flow into the Gulf of Mexico. The *desagüe* of Huehuetoca took only ten months to complete (29 November 1607 to 17 September 1608), and more than sixty thousand Indians were employed with losses of only ten or twenty dead from illness. Ten died following accidents and fifty-three due to illness endemic to the area of Huehuetoca. Its initial cost was three hundred thousand pesos, a sum that represented seventeen percent of the American silver that the Crown received as an annual average between 1606 and 1610, and fifteen per cent of the annual average income of the Royal Treasury of Mexico City.[8] However, after 1608, the drainage of Huchuetoca was neither properly maintained nor enlarged, and engineer Enrico Martínez,[9] the author of the project, faced both technical and financial problems. The entire project was definitively halted in 1623 due to the conflicts that arose within the different government branches responsible for urban affairs.[10] The complete halt of the *desagüe* led to the most serious flood the city had experienced in its history, the flood of 1629. The rain began to pour down on the day of Saint Matthew, 21 September, and its persistence was such that it kept the city under water until 1634. During those years, more than thirty thousand people died from drowning, illness and/or hunger, and of the twenty thousand families who inhabited the city in 1629, only four hundred remained by 1634, since many of those who managed to flee established themselves in Puebla.[11] In 1629, one eyewitness, the Dominican friar Alonso Franco, described the city as a vast shipwreck:

> ... her houses and churches though of stone, looked more like ships than buildings, which rested on the earth. They seemed to be floating upon the water, and as with waterlogged ships, which need to pump incessantly, in the houses and churches the pumping went on day and night.[12]

In 1630, due to the chaotic situation, the Church, officials and engineers proposed a number of alternative projects. One involved abandoning the city and rebuilding it in a safer site, a proposal supported in 1630–31 by Archbishop Manso and by the King of Spain, but opposed by Viceroy Cerralvo and by many inhabitants of the city.[13] Another proposal, made by the Jesuit priest Francisco Calderón, involved searching for a mythical *sumidero,* a "natural tunnel reputed to lie in Lake Texcoco that had consumed the flood waters during Aztec times."[14] With the help of three hundred Indians, the search began in 1631, but the *sumidero* was never found. The need to find a solution to the problem was urgent: the city was completely swamped, many people feared the outbreak of epidemics, and even though it was a question of debate whether the enclosed chain of lakes, "the evil stepmother of this city" (in Hoberman's phrase), were intrinsically unhealthy, what was agreed upon was that floods caused illness and death.[15] Another project put forward at the time by Simón Méndez involved building a canal that would drain Lake Texcoco directly and therefore prevent the back flow of its water into the city. However, to do this, that is, to build the so-called "universal drainage system" (*desagüe universal*), would involve an enormous expenditure of time, money and men, and it was cheaper, safer and easier, financially and politically, to continue with the *desagüe* of Huehuetoca. Thus, when the works resumed in 1637, it was decided that the tunnel would be converted into an open trench that would serve to carry off the water of the river Cuautitlán and remove one of the chief causes of flooding. It was thought that an open trench would bring an end to the blockages that could occur in the tunnel. However, what was not realized was that erosion would continue unless the sides of the open canal were given a gentle slope.[16]

The works on the *desagüe* continued from 1607 until 1789, in particular during times of crisis, when floods threatened the livelihood of the inhabitants of the city and the city itself, as occurred in 1645, 1674, 1691, 1707, 1714, 1724, 1747 and 1763. When the *desagüe* of Huehuetoca was officially "perfected" in 1789, it proved that what was required was to drain Lake Texcoco, as Simón Méndez had indicated in March 1630. Otherwise, the danger of the lake rising and flooding the city during the season of heavy rain would remain a menace to the city and its inhabitants.[17]

In 1902, historian Luis González Obregón argued that work on the *desagüe* had consumed more than seven million pesos between 1607 and 1822, and that experience had shown that in order to free the city from floods it was necessary to establish long-term continuity in the works, economic resources and labour, and an efficient administrative apparatus exclusively devoted to the *desagüe*.[18] What was required was a centralized administration and a permanent bureaucracy. During the course of the nineteenth century, the problems caused by floods within the capital continued: the city was seriously flooded in 1819, 1856, 1865 and 1894, and the issue of the *desagüe* became a national obsession as the century progressed. This led many politicians, engineers and physicians, regardless of their political orientation, to put forward proposals and projects in order to find a definitive solution to a problem that had accompanied the city throughout its history. Lucas Alamán was keenly interested and wrote in 1823 about this public work; and politician José María Luis Mora visited the drainage of Huehuetoca in 1823 and wrote a report on its condition.[19] Even Alexander Von Humboldt, during his trips across New Spain in 1803 and 1804, spent time inspecting and writing about the drainage works.[20] However, it was only after the 1856 flood that the issue of the drainage system was seriously considered once again, as the unsanitary conditions led to the outbreak of both epidemic and non-epidemic diseases. The reasons for the neglect of the *desagüe* between 1821 and 1856 were numerous, among them the constant political upheavals experienced by the country after Independence, the scarcity of economic resources and the lack of continuity in the administration of the project, as there was no single branch of government exclusively devoted to the *desagüe*.[21]

This latter problem was solved in April 1853, when the government created the Ministry of Development (Secretaría de Fomento). Among the obligations faced by this ministry, whose name itself points towards the idea of "progress," was the task of administering and promoting the *desagüe* of the city and valley of Mexico. In 1856, the Minister of Development, Manuel Siliceo, appointed a commission composed of politicians and engineers to reconsider the whole subject of the *desagüe*, and offered a prize of twelve thousand pesos to the best project for effectively draining the valley so that the city might be free of danger from floods.[22] Six projects were presented, and that of engineer Francisco de Garay was accepted. This project planned to carry off the surplus water of the lakes and the sewage of the city by means of a canal (Gran Canal), a tunnel and an outflow ditch. The Gran Canal would start at the southeast end of the city, in the Barrio de San Lázaro, and pass through lakes Texcoco, San Cristóbal, Xaltocan and Zumpango. The total length of the Gran Canal would be more than forty-seven kilometres. Between the end of the Gran Canal and the beginning of the tunnel, a reservoir to control the amount of water flowing into the tunnel would be built. The tunnel would be more than ten kilometres long, and all the water flowing through it would reach an outflow ditch of 2.5 kilometres. This outflow ditch would lead the water into a tributary of the river Tula, the river Pánuco, and finally all the water would be expelled into the Gulf of Mexico (see Figure 6).[23]

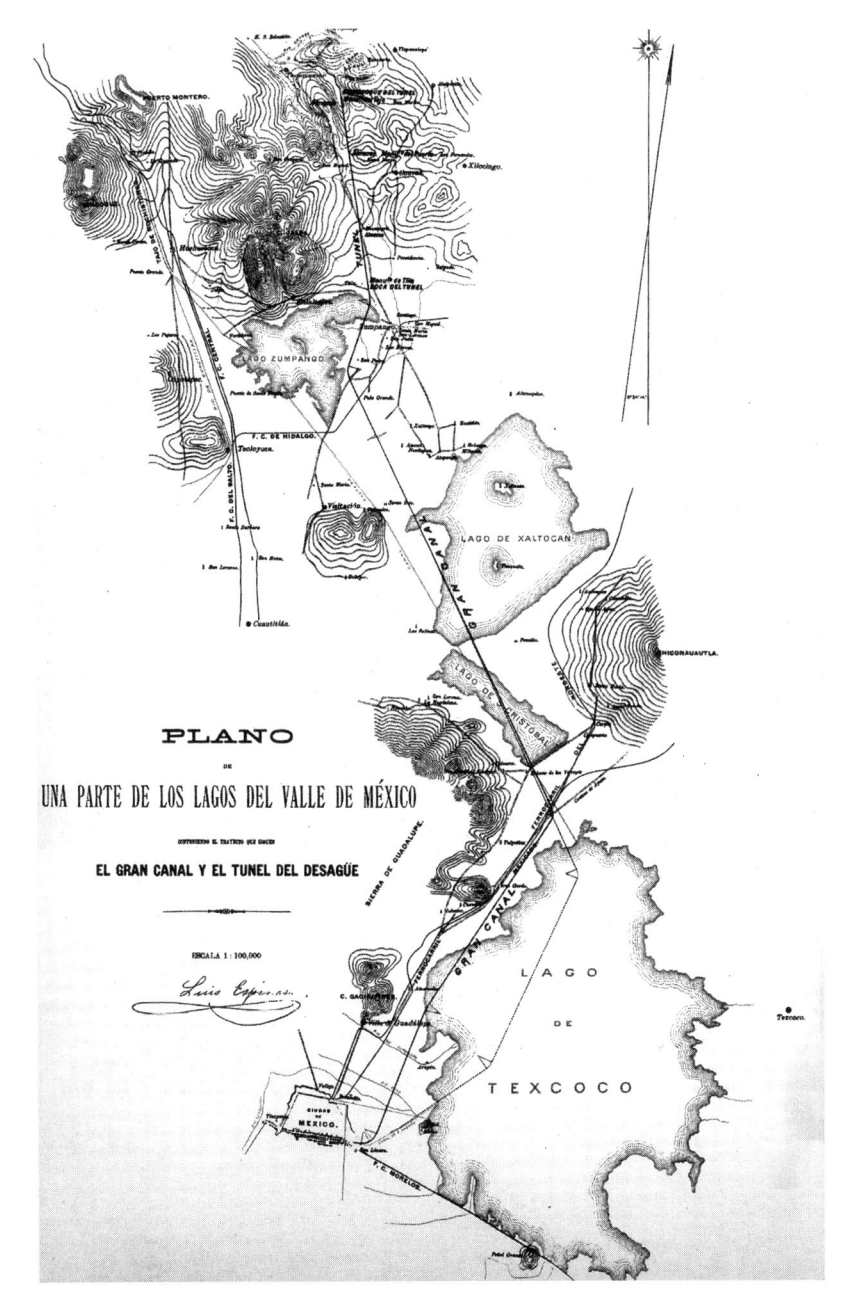

Figure 6. Map of the Lakes in the Valley of Mexico, of the Gran Canal and of the Tunnel of the Desagüe.
© Archivo Histórico del Agua, Mexico. Photograph by Alex Larrondo.

It was thought that this project, when completed as outlined above, would at last control the disruptions caused to the city by flooding, and epidemic and non-epidemic disease would be prevented by flushing away the waste before it rotted into dangerous miasmas. This project, formally inaugurated in March 1900 by Porfirio Díaz, symbolized the triumph of science and technology, presenting an optimistic view of how technical solutions could be devised to control the city and, by extension, how technical solutions could also be applied to solve public health issues.[24]

The Drainage System

As the previous pages have shown, the attempts to deal with the problems caused by excess water had as long a history as the city, and during the Porfiriato, doctors, engineers and the government not only set about offering a definitive solution to these problems, but also wrote detailed studies of how the city drainage system had been constructed at different historical periods, with what materials and techniques and with what degree of effectiveness. For instance, in 1901 a study was made expressly for the delegates of the Pan-American Congress held in Mexico City, and was entitled *Brief Sketch of the Drainage Works of the Valley of Mexico*. This study, as its title indicates, presented a historical summary of the drainage problems the city had suffered from its foundation as Tenochtitlán until the government of Porfirio Díaz, and emphasized that finally, following the advances in science and technology and the political stability and economic development made possible by the Díaz government, the city was to become a safe and prosperous place to live.[25]

However, the most important book written during the Porfiriato that dealt with all these issues was the monumental *Memoria histórica, técnica y administrativa de las obras del desagüe del Valle de México, 1449–1900,* published by the Junta Directiva de las Obras del Desagüe in 1902. The *Memoria* included detailed studies by prominent engineers and historians of the time. Historian Luis González Obregón dealt with the historical aspect of the works, and also wrote the general introduction; engineers Luis Espinosa and Isidro Díaz Lombardo reviewed the technical aspects of the construction of the drainage system, while engineer Rosendo Esparza analyzed its administrative and financial aspects.[26] This monumental work clearly shows that the

Porfirian administration regarded the *desagüe* as one of its most important priorities and as a public work that would free the city from the almost eternal threat of floods. The *desagüe* became the symbol of what good administration, technical knowledge and careful investigation could accomplish at a time of increased wealth, peace and prosperity.

Engineer Espinosa argued that during Díaz's first term in office (1877–80), most measures taken to prevent the overflow of the city's sewers and canals relied on keeping them free of obstructions, and that due to the lack of adequate drainage and sewer systems, the sanitary condition of the city relied upon the hope that the city's inhabitants would follow the numerous hygienic regulations laid down to keep the city clean.[27]

However, the cleansing of the city was not enough to restrain the invasion of water, and the Minister of Development, Vicente Riva Palacio believed that the drainage system, when completed, would deliver the benefits everyone had sought for so long.[28] The previous chapters have shown that most measures advanced by public health officials to improve the unsanitary conditions of the city emphasized the need to keep the city clean, to clear, cover and drain all open ditches and sewers, to sweep streets and clean public fountains, among other things. In 1881, the Superior Sanitation Council stated through one of its commissions that in order to prevent a health crisis, particular attention should be given to its sewers, and recommended that all of them should be cleansed, that no animal or human waste should be thrown into them and that the police should ensure that the measures were followed, particularly in tenement buildings. It added that the best time of day to clean the sewers was at night or very early in the morning, before the heat of the sun caused the evaporation of the tainted water, causing the spread of sources of infection. The Superior Sanitation Council also believed that the miasmas could be destroyed by burning the deposits of stagnant materials and by the use of disinfectants.[29]

The concern about unsanitary conditions in the capital and the incidence of premature death, in particular among children, was also highlighted in 1882. On 21 January, the Congreso Higiénico Pedagógico was inaugurated in the capital, and one of the topics discussed was the importance of education and adequate schools for the development of hygienic practices among children. In 1883, the first Congreso Nacional de Higiene was also held in Mexico City; this analyzed the possible measures that could be taken to upgrade the sanitary conditions of the nation and to prevent epidemic diseases from entering the country via its ports and borders.[30] The recommendations made by the Superior Sanitation Council in 1881 and by the congresses held in 1882 and 1883 pointed to the growing distaste for dirt and increased concern for public health at a time when the city was expanding at an unprecedented rate. At the same time as physicians and hygienists were gathering to discuss what could be done to improve the sanitary conditions of the capital, engineers drew up projects for the best sewer and drainage system they could think of.

Floods and infection caused architect and civil engineer Ricardo Orozco to submit a project to the Commission of Public Works in 1884, and to establish that those were the "great evils" the capital faced. He argued that the problem of floods was not exclusive to Mexico, and that in Holland the authorities continually had to devise methods to contain water and prevent floods. The Dutch had successfully managed to do so by building dikes and by pumping out water, but this method, he argued, was not appropriate for Mexico City. With regard to the infection caused by putrefying waste and stagnant water, the only solution known to be efficient, and also to prevent floods, relied on a drainage system.[31]

Unlike cities such as London, Paris and New York, located next to rivers into which they could channel waste water, Mexico City had the disadvantage of being located in an unfortunate geographical site. It had no large rivers and was surrounded by mountains within an enclosed valley. Engineer Orozco argued that it was in those major cities that the most adequate sanitary measures had been implemented, and that after a very careful study of how they had dealt with or were dealing with their sanitary problems, he had reached the conclusion that the only real solution for Mexico City was the drainage of the city. The drainage of the city and valley of Mexico would solve the problem of floods, but he conceived the drainage system as the "complement" of the sewer system.[32]

Engineer Orozco's project was based on the belief that it was imperative to lower the water level of the city and to provide sufficient movement in the sewers to avoid stagnation. But this measure would be useless unless the city were properly drained, by means of a Gran Canal to expel all water – both rain and waste water. And this, he was certain, could be accomplished.[33]

The arguments in favour of the *desagüe* were also shared by the journal of the Municipal Council, and its adherence to the proposal was based on the impact that this public work would have on the health of the capital.

In an article published on 22 July 1885, *El Municipio Libre* categorically affirmed that the only possible way to prevent a cholera epidemic from invading not only the capital but the entire country was to drain all visible water, marshes and swamps, to plant as many trees as possible, to provide abundant drinking water to all towns and cities, and to establish good public services for the collection of rubbish and waste.[34]

Thus, by the mid-1880s, after many years of deliberations, projects and proposals, it was widely believed that the drainage system that should be built was the same that had been proposed by engineer Francisco de Garay in 1856, a project which had been perfected by engineer Luis Espinosa during the 1870s, and which engineer Ricardo Orozco had revived in 1884. It was also thought that the drainage system could be successfully completed in the climate of political stability and social peace present in the country, and this had a great deal to do with the increasingly strong and interventionist role of a state that aimed to create a thoroughly modern Mexico.

After General Manuel González's interregnum as President of the Republic (1880–84), Porfirio Díaz secured his position as President, a position he was not to abandon until his resignation in 1911. In 1885, in a meeting between Díaz and the President of the Municipal Council, General Pedro Rincón Gallardo, and the Regidor de Obras Públicas, engineer Manuel María Contreras, it was decided that the drainage works must go ahead in order to improve the sanitary conditions in the city, and that therefore the Municipal Council would allocate two hundred thousand pesos per year to the task. In the opinion of Porfirio Díaz, the drainage system was nothing other than a public health work.[35]

The drainage works would guarantee not only the prosperity of the capital city, but also the health of its inhabitants. In 1886, after Díaz's visit to the "public health work," he submitted a proposal to Congress that involved allocating an annual sum not of two hundred thousand but of four hundred thousand pesos for the construction of this public work. Additionally, a loan was secured from London (£2,400,000) that was to be exclusively used for the *desagüe*. Thus the project had been approved, and it was financially safe to proceed, but it was also essential to have the full co-operation of specialists in engineering, public health and sanitation. To fill this void, the Junta Directiva del Desagüe del Valle de México was created on 9 February 1886. The director of the Junta Directiva was engineer Luis Espinosa; the Ministry of Development was responsible for the technical aspects of the public works, and its president was the leader of the Municipal Council, Pedro Rincón Gallardo. The Junta Directiva also included Jose Yves Limantour, Agustín Cerdan, Francisco Rivas Góngora, Pablo Macedo, Gabriel Mancera and Rosendo Esparza, among others.[36] The Junta Directiva became a bureaucracy staffed by skilled experts with a long-term commitment, and during the official inauguration of the Junta Directiva, Rincón Gallardo stated the following:

> By special order from the President of the Republic, who has seen with great pleasure the zeal with which you wish to carry out the important public work to give health and life to our unhealthy city ... you will have the satisfaction of having assured for yourself and your descendants man's most valuable good — health — seriously imperiled by the dirtiness of this city. Moreover, your names will go on to posterity, overflowing with blessings, not only from the Mexicans who will be saved from illnesses, premature death and the ruin of their properties, but by the whole Republic, interested in the resurgence of our beautiful capital.[37]

In July 1886, five months after the Junta Directiva had been officially inaugurated and the *desagüe* praised as a public work that would bring health to the city, health to the inhabitants, and glory to those responsible for such a historic task, the newspaper *El Tiempo* made critical comments when a storm flooded many central streets, stressing the fact that instead of terrestrial vehicles, the inhabitants required canoes to go from one place to the other.[38] Press criticisms proliferated every time the city was flooded, and some articles argued that the Municipal Council was more concerned with embellishing the city by introducing historical monuments, gardens and ornate fountains than with finding a definitive solution to a problem that threatened the health of the inhabitants.[39] The complaints were not only expressed in the press. Many inhabitants wrote to the Municipal Council, demanding not only a prompt solution but also compensation for the damage caused to their houses and/or businesses by floods. In a letter written in 1888 to the Municipal

Council, Mr. Mariano Panes argued that his home and surrounding property had become flooded and demanded compensation for the damage caused. The reply he received from the government stated that the authorities were not responsible for the losses Mr. Panes had suffered, and that he would therefore receive no compensation.[40] In 1893, the owner of the textile factory *La Victoria*, located in the eastern part of the city very close to the Canal de la Viga, argued that all his employees had to do their duties with water up to their knees, adding that the Canal de la Viga rose 8.65 metres, flooding the entire barrio of La Resurrección.[41] The Municipal Council also received another letter in 1897, signed by a Mr. Tiburcio Olmos, who requested compensation of 825 pesos for a flood that caused the collapse of seven of the thirty-three rooms he had built to let to the poorest people of the city. According to Mr. Olmos, the force of the water was such that it had been impossible to contain it. The Municipal Council sent engineer Esparza to assess what had caused the collapse of the rooms, and his report stated that the rooms were built with poor quality materials, that they lacked firm foundations and that it would have been unsafe to rent them. Therefore, there was no reason why Mr. Olmos should be given the compensation he requested.[42]

In the midst of the wave of criticisms and demands made by the inhabitants of the city, the Junta Directiva began to work in 1886 under the leadership of engineer Espinosa, who said that the public works had the following objectives and characteristics: first, to prevent floods; second, to receive all tainted water from Mexico City and drive it out of the Valley; and third, to "govern" water, in particular the water that was harmful to health. The public works would have three main parts: a Canal, a Tunnel and an Outflow Ditch.[43] The aim was no less than the conquest of water. Of the three key elements mentioned by Espinosa, only the outflow ditch was almost finished, because it had been dug between 1868 and 1870.[44] The tunnel and the canal were the most difficult and required much more work, money and time than the outflow ditch. And by 1889, due to technical, administrative and organizational inefficiency, as well as the lack of machinery and dredges, Mr. José Yves Limantour argued that it was necessary to resort to foreign help.[45]

The need to seek foreign assistance also stemmed from another problem mentioned by Limantour, namely "the character of our people." Because of the supposedly inherent deficiencies of the national character, it was imperative to seek the advice of special men who "have acquired enough experience in similar tasks, and that have the tenacity and spirit to see through tasks of this nature, surpassing all difficulties be them technical or economic."[46] Advice had been sought in British and United States engineering firms for the construction of railways, for Mexico City's tramways and in mines, and the contract for the *desagüe* tunnel was initially given to the company Read and Campbell of London, and the contract for the Gran Canal to the American Dredging Company. However, these contracts were cancelled after the works saw no major progress, and other foreign engineering firms were sought. The task of building the Gran Canal — the core of the drainage system — was given to the British firm Pearson and Sons, led by Sir Weetman Pearson (later Lord Cowdray). When the contract was signed by Romero Rubio and Pearson and Sons on 23 December 1889, it stated that the Junta Directiva of the Desagüe would deliver to the Contractor, with the least possible delay, the lands required for both for the excavation of the Canal and the side banks.[47] This meant that through the construction of the *desagüe*, the city would expand and would claim or appropriate all land required for this public work. Through the *desagüe*, the countryside would be transformed as a result of the use of machinery, organized labour and foreign expertise for the benefit of the capital city. The construction of this major public work ignored municipal and state boundaries and followed the natural gradients of the terrain to achieve the incline required to expel all waste from the city (see Figure 7).

According to John Body, general manager of Pearson and Sons in Mexico, the drainage works had two major objectives: first, to control the level of the lakes and waters of the valley; and second, to receive the sewage of the city of Mexico and carry the whole of it outside the valley.[48] The resources invested in the *desagüe* between February 1886 and June 1900 amounted to 15,967,778 pesos, and the work on the Gran Canal begun in January 1890 was largely concluded by June 1896. However, the entire drainage work was not completed until 1900. During its construction, there was continuous surveillance of the workers, with fines for those who did not work efficiently, and labour was organized in three shifts of eight hours each. The excavation of the Gran Canal to a depth sufficient to float the dredgers was done manually (4,800,000 cubic metres), a process which Mr. Body described as follows:

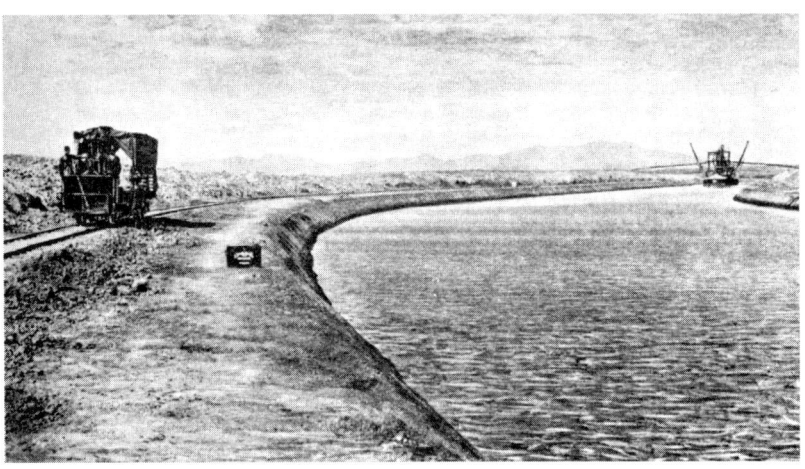

Figure 7. The Gran Canal of Desagüe, 1900.
© Archivo Histórico del Agua, Mexico. Photograph by Alex Larrondo.

This work was done by Indians by task-work, the earth being removed to a distance of about 100 feet, in a rough net or basket carried on the back and supported by a strap from the head, each man carrying and digging alternately. The Indians execute all kinds of earthworks very satisfactorily provided that sufficient care is taken to keep the work to proper time and level.[49]

Railways were used to transport most of the necessary materials and equipment, and the main administrative and technical offices were located in the town of Zumpango, which became known as the "capital" of the drainage works. Because of the extension of the drainage works, it became necessary to build aqueduct-bridges for rivers and canals, bridges for railroads and for other terrestrial vehicles.[50] At first there was only one doctor at the site, but due to the accidents that inevitably occurred, a hospital was built exclusively for those working on the *desagüe*. When fatal accidents took place, the Junta Directiva gave the family of the deceased compensation equal to the work the victim had accomplished, but also considered whether incompetence or carelessness had had any bearing on the accident before giving the money to the family.[51]

With the *desagüe*, the overflow of Lake Texcoco would be controlled, restraining the invasion of tainted water into the city. However, in order to attain the health, order and cleanliness of the city, in particular by eradicating the overflow and putrid stenches arising from its sewers, what was required was the rebuilding of the entire sewage system.

The Sewage System

In 1888, the Municipal Council decided that an urgent overhaul of the city's inefficient sewers was required, and to this end created the Junta de las Obras de Saneamiento de la Ciudad de México, a commission of engineers whose task was to compile all the relevant information in order to proceed. After three years of careful study, the results were given to engineers Luis Espinosa, Manuel Contreras, Leandro Fernández and Roberto Gayol, who studied the information and assessed which would be the best sewage system for the capital.

The situation the city's sewers faced was as follows: they were primarily storm sewers, and their main function was rainwater drainage, but they were also used for the disposal of waste water, both from factories and houses. Sewers were of three types: underground, open sewers and gutters. However, many open sewers and gutters were also used to dispose of human and animal waste. The liquid waste was meant to flow into the underground sewers, then into the Canal de San Lázaro, and finally into Lake Texcoco. However, because the underground sewers were generally clogged, whenever the city flooded following a heavy rainfall or the overflow of Lake Texcoco, all the sewers also overflowed. It is not surprising that due to their inefficiency during those years it was said that it was best to try to imagine than to describe the state of the subsoil under the city. Such unsanitary conditions led to a mortality rate that reached forty per thousand, and it was thought that the city had the highest mortality rate in the civilized world. It was also argued that the only factor that protected the city to some degree from pestilence was its altitude of over seven thousand feet above sea level, but that nonetheless, malarial and gastric fevers were almost endemic.[52] According to Matías Romero, the problem of the drainage system was one that for a century "has been settling into one of pure sanitation."[53] Although the government had called for plans for draining the valley, what was really needed was to dispose of the sewage. The drainage system was thus to be simply a part of the sewage system of the city.

When the project for the new sewage system was made public by engineer Roberto Gayol in 1895, its aim was to take advantage of the drainage system being built and to take all the waste water into the drainage system and out of the city. The sewage system proposed was then known as a "combined sewage system."[54] This type of system was also used in Paris, Berlin, Brussels, Vienna and New York, examples that had been carefully studied by Gayol, Espinosa and other engineers.[55] The combined system was intended to have a large enough capacity to receive all domestic waste, and the volume of precipitation it would have to cope with suggested that the network had to be colossal in scale, and that the rubbish collected from street sweeping should never enter the system. A major problem facing this type of sewage system was the lack of sufficient water to maintain movement at all times and thus to cleanse the network, a problem that could arise in times of drought or when it became clogged, causing the accumulated deposits to ferment. However, it was not only the decaying organic matter that could cause disease; some doctors believed that the sewers could exude an odourless gas that caused innumerable infectious and non-infectious diseases.

The construction of the new sewage system did not begin until 1897, and between 1888 and 1897, the National Academy of Medicine and the Superior Sanitation Council made detailed studies of the impact the new public work would have on the health of the city and its inhabitants. In 1893, the Superior Sanitation Council made a number of recommendations to be followed in the city to prevent the development of a typhus epidemic. Among them was the building of a new sewage system, and the Council emphasized the aspects to be avoided if the system adopted was the "combined system": deficient ventilation and the stagnation of water. The lack of ventilation, according to the members of the Academy of Medicine, caused two serious problems: waste water produced miasmas, and the products of this decomposition led to the proliferation of germs; and both miasmas and germs were taken into all houses causing disease.[56] The reference made to both miasmas and germs points to the fact that the initial understandings of the germ theory "were deeply indebted to an older scientific discipline, that is, to sanitary science, which stressed the ubiquity of airborne infection and the disease-causing properties of human wastes, organic decay" — and miasmas.[57] In another study carried out in

1896 by the Hygiene Commission of the National Academy of Medicine, it expressed to the Comisión de Obras Públicas the view that the entire sewer system had to be rebuilt (otherwise the drainage system would be useless), and that the new sewers should be built at the same time as the drainage works.[58] Some members of the National Academy of Medicine believed that the main cause of premature death among the urban population was the proliferation of infectious diseases, and these, they argued, had their origin in the impregnation of the soil, land and water with putrefying organic waste. It was therefore necessary to drain the land, to install adequate sewers and to take all waste and excess water out of the city.[59]

Physicians were of the opinion that only some African cities had a higher mortality rate than Mexico City, and the causes mentioned included the lack of drinking water, inefficient sewers and waste-disposal systems, as well as the dirt found in many streets. Another origin of the problem was to be found in the misery, poverty and vice of large sectors of the urban poor.[60] The link between misery, poverty and vice among the urban population and the lack of water was repeatedly stressed at the time. It was upheld by the belief that the majority of the population, due to their lack of education and superstitious behaviour, lived in crowded and unsanitary conditions. Most Mexicans, it was assumed, were ignorant, did not have any sentiments of true citizenship, resorted to magic and quacks when ill, and loved to drink but not to work.[61] Therefore, the efforts of the government to attain a clean and hygienic city were continuously boycotted and thwarted because of the popular customs of its inhabitants.[62] The Mexican people had to be educated and to learn the principles of hygiene and morality if the city was to be transformed. This process would take some time; in the meantime, the cleansing of the city had to go ahead.

The doctors of the National Academy of Medicine thought that it was important to build the drainage and sewers simultaneously, so that the overall sanitation would be less expensive and also because of their theory that digging up the streets brought pathogenic germs and miasmas into contact with the air, and that if this happened, they would become more dangerous and their circulation within the city on air currents would be enhanced.[63] This again points to the fact that the miasmatic theory of disease remained entrenched in public health thinking and that the germ theory of disease to a large degree reinforced the assumptions of the environmental theories by confirming the risks of polluted air and water. This opinion was shared by the members of the Superior Sanitation Council, when it expressed in 1897 that it was crucial to provide constant movement to the water below the city, to avoid the stagnation and decay of all waste in order to prevent the creation of sites of decomposition and miasmatic emanations.[64]

Other proposals made during those years to reduce the danger posed to public health by water, land and atmospheric pollution caused by sewers and open ditches favoured the use of charcoal and other chemical disinfectants.[65] In 1881, Dr. Huerta stated that he was convinced that the use of disinfectants would lead to the eradication of noxious odours, and that this was an inexpensive, practical and easy method of dealing with urgent health problems.[66] However, his proposal was rejected by Dr. Nicolás Ramírez de Arellano, a prominent member of the Superior Sanitation Council, who replied that only sanitary science, that is the drainage and sewage systems, would remove all human and animal waste from the city, and that only then would Lake Texcoco cease to be the cesspool of the capital.[67] Arellano also stressed that agriculture would benefit from waste water if it were used as a fertilizer. Thus, the conversion of sewage into fertilizer would render a threat invisible and would transform it into a benefit to both the city and the countryside. If urban waste could be used for agriculture in the regions surrounding the city, a balance between the city and the countryside could be achieved. The aim was to pump clean or pure water from the countryside into the city, and to evacuate the city's waste into the countryside, where it could be of use and transform arid regions into arable land. The importance of recycling urban waste was medical, economic and a matter of human survival. In France, during the mid-nineteenth century, as Alain Corbin has shown, engineer A. Mille held that "every unpleasant odor signals a blow to public health in the towns, and a loss of manure in the countryside."[68] Arellano also believed that the transfer of sewage was a priority.

The combined sewer system was intended to receive household sewage and rain water from particular areas of the city (the most modern *colonias*); this waste water would be brought to each of the five main sewers located in the city and would then be pumped into pipes leading out of the city and into the Gran Canal del Desagüe.[69] Special care had to be taken to avoid dead ends within the system because they constituted foci of infection. The continual flushing of the sewers would guarantee their permanent good order and cleanliness. The water was to be taken from the Canal de la Viga and by means of sudden rushes of water the liquid would flow through the sewers. Mexico City's sewer system would accomplish what no other system in the world had managed to do, to flush every day all the sewers of the city. The construction of manholes and lamp-holes would allow for their inspection and the removal of any accidental obstacle with the greatest of ease and without digging up the sewers or the paving of the streets. In times of drought or other unfortunate situations, "a gang of twenty men would be enough to clean the sewers everyday."[70]

Porfirio Díaz, in his address to Congress in September 1903, stated that sanitary conditions in the capital continued to improve, and in particular he emphasized the role sewers had played.[71] The sewage system was formally inaugurated in 1905, and according to Pablo Macedo, its cost up to 1903, without taking into consideration the additional expense of re-paving the city's streets, amounted to 8,043,616 pesos.[72] According to Matías Romero, both the sewage and drainage systems would transform the city into one of the healthiest in the world, its inhabitants would have more security, enjoy longer lives, prosperity would increase, and

> the population will grow rapidly, not to mention the tide of tourists that will set in from the Unites States, and this will mean larger revenues for the municipality. So after a weary search of centuries for relief, the beautiful Valley of Mexico will gain its deliverance not only from the engulfing floods, but also from the sanitary evils that have long resulted from defective drainage.[73]

During the construction of the sewage system, there were numerous claims and remarks by the inhabitants about the chaos the construction caused in the city's streets, making it dangerous to circulate within them. Some inhabitants feared that the excavations required to install the sewers would damage the foundations of their homes and cause their collapse. In October 1889, a group of neighbours whose houses were located near an area where one of the main sewers was to be built wrote to the Municipal Council saying that they feared the collapse of their homes if the excavations proceeded. In January 1900, the Municipal Council replied, underlining that it was useless to discuss the importance or convenience the public works had, and added that the inquiries carried out by the Municipal Council proved that the city's inhabitants had no good reason to be afraid.[74] In March 1900, the newspaper *El Imparcial* argued that the material progress of the city was becoming more evident as the days went by, and told its readers that the removal of pavements and the obstruction of the streets were nothing other than proofs that all civilized centres had to overcome if they were to become sites of well-being for their inhabitants. Even though the sanitation works caused annoyance to the population — it added — they would benefit the health and living conditions of all citizens. Therefore, the article urged the urban population to support and work towards the health of the city and to understand that the chaotic situation was ultimately in the best interests of the city.[75] But a guide to Mexico City warned its readers of the chaos to be found in the city's streets:

> … many residents of Mexico have died victims of infectious diseases contracted as a result of the fetid and foul-smelling emanations from the sewers and open ditches in the streets and squares for the drainage works; others have fallen to the ground … breaking their head or ribs at the mercy of the invasion of the slippery slime thrown onto the sidewalks by the drainage workers … Other good residents … if they have had the fortune of not being blind or short sighted, or of not walking at night with the lack of balance which an immoderate use of alcohol causes in the legs (in both cases they run the imminent risk of taking a bath of foul-smelling water and of filth at the bottom of the open sewers), in order to arrive at a place just six or seven streets away … are forced to make a thousand detours to avoid the clogged, flooded and infected places …[76]

Regardless of the criticisms, demands and complaints articulated by some inhabitants of the city about the construction of the public works, and regardless of the indifference that others felt towards the idea of a hygienic city, the construction of the public works was too important to the government, engineers and public health officials for it to be suspended.

During the final decades of the nineteenth century, the city was incessantly described and dissected, and its underground was repeatedly explored. The metaphor of the city as a diseased organism or living body implied that it required a thorough investigation and classification of all its ills, efficient co-ordination and organization to restore its condition, and that it was crucial to give free circulation to its subsoil. The underground — the invisible — was unveiled, the movement of water had to be controlled and the threats emanating from the sewers eliminated. The biological metaphors used to describe the city were also employed for its social problems or social diseases, among which alcoholism and prostitution stood out. For instance, Dr. Luis Lara y Pardo wrote in 1908 that science had clearly proven that prostitution was a degenerative state of social and psychological inferiority and a threat to educated people, as he commented in his book *La prostitución en México*.[77] The statistical information gathered by the sanitary inspectors and used by Lara y Pardo suggested that the city had 10,937 registered prostitutes in 1904; 11,554 in 1905; and 9,742 in 1906. Moreover, Lara y Pardo acknowledged that to make matters worse, the figures were not even exact and that they did not include clandestine prostitutes.[78]

Even though this book does not deal with either prostitution or alcoholism during the Porfiriato, it is important to consider an interesting description of the city's sewers found in the novel *Santa*, written by Federico Gamboa, and published in 1903.[79] The book narrates the life of Santa, a beautiful peasant girl who, after being seduced by a military man from the city, had no option but to flee her town — Chimalistac — after her besmirched honour and name brought shame to her and her family. In the city, she was corrupted by the vices and immorality of the Capital; she engaged in prostitution, having no other option, and died of cervical cancer. Lara y Pardo explicitly criticized Gamboa's novel by stating that romantic novels had transformed the figure of the prostitute into a heroine, particularly in countries with a Latin temperament.[80] And when Gamboa described the immorality and diseased condition of Santa, who was close to death, he did so by evoking images of the sewers. It must be noted that the thorough investigation of both sewers and prostitution was undertaken in France by the hygienist Alexandre Parent-Duchâtelet during the 1830s, and that his studies must have been known in Mexico, as reference to him is continuously made by Lara y Pardo.[81] It is possible that Gamboa was acquainted with Parent-Duchâtelet's studies, but what is certain is that in his novels he attempted to present extreme cases of modern life in the capital.[82] The image Gamboa presents is the following:

> Santa descended, downwards, always further down ... a superhuman force has cast her to drift with formidable drive through all the murkiness of the bottomless heights of the enormous corrupted city. Santa drifted through this murkiness, in the pestilent basements, black from inferior vice, she drifted in the same way as the dirty and impure waters from the subterranean sewers angrily gallop through the dark intestines of the streets, with a sinister glug-glug of imprisoned liquid that has to flow in an invariable direction even though it is opposed, even though it swirls around in corners and suspicious and foul-smelling cavities, places which those above do not know of ... There goes the water, unknowable, without crystals on its back, without freshness in its lymph; transporting detritus and microbes, all that which stinks and kills; portraying the black, the hidden, the unnamed that should not be revealed; emitting through every vent of the grating, a heavy reek, an anguished and hoarse murmur of exhaustion, of sadness, of sorrow ... there it goes, ejected from the city and from the people, to pound against the irons of the exit, to die at sea, which shrouds it and protects it, perhaps it is only the sea that remembers that it was born pure; in the mountain, quenching the thirst and fertilizing the fields, that it was dew, perfume, life ...[83]

Gamboa depicts the irreversible moral and physical downfall of Santa, and the figure of the prostitute is metamorphosed into a sewer, a site of decomposition, disease and contagion which takes hold of the city.

Both the sewers and the prostitute belonged to the underground, to the intestines of the streets, and their corrupted and dangerous liquids and stenches harmed and killed. The final and only solution was their eradication from the city: death for the prostitute, and the sea for the sewage. The unnamable and unknowable became the sites of social investigation by public health officials. Gamboa's description of the repugnant and corrupted elements of urban life was influenced by the topographical investigations or diagnoses of the city made during the final decades of the nineteenth century, and also by the impact naturalism had in late –nineteenth century Mexican literature. Gamboa also presented a clear opposition between the countryside and city, through which he idealized rural areas.

The idealization of the countryside took place at a time when increased urbanization led many to regard the capital as a site of corruption, danger, filth and moral degeneration.[84] The city was thought to be particularly dangerous for women and their fulfilment of the duty that society and nature had entrusted them with: to be respectable mothers, wives and daughters.[85] However, the fact that Gamboa resorted to the city's sewers to portray the inevitable death of Santa also points to the fact that he used a problematical element of the city of which most inhabitants were well aware, and which could be easily remembered, evoked, seen and smelled.

The official optimism that had accompanied the construction of the drainage and sewage works became manifest during their inauguration. During the month of March 1900, most of the capital's newspapers began to prepare the limited reading public for an event without precedent in the history of the city. On 16 March 1900, *El Imparcial* began its report on the inauguration of the drainage works by stating that it was possible that many of its readers were not fully aware of the astounding magnitude of the project and the huge problems they would solve, adding that the threat of floods would disappear, that the city would finally be a healthy environment, with no bad odours or filth; that the flow of sewage out of the city would increase the region's agricultural production and that it would also be used for the production of hydroelectric power.[86] The success of the public works could not have been greater, and the chronicles of the event itself magnified this optimism.

On the morning of Saturday, 17 March 1900, the city was awakened by the sound of all the church bells announcing the inauguration of the drainage works.[87] The sound of the bells, the music of victory in war, notified the entire population that a secular struggle had finally been won. On that morning, General Porfirio Díaz and a select group of 180 guests (including all the members of the Junta Directiva de las Obras del Desagüe, the diplomatic body and government representatives) met at eight o'clock at the Palacio Nacional where ten special vehicles took them to San Lázaro, the focal point of celebration. General Porfirio Díaz formally inaugurated the public works at nine o'clock.[88] An achievement that no other government in the history of the city had managed to attain was celebrated in a public ceremony that included a select group of men and excluded the majority of the urban population, just as the public works had.

Pedro Rincón Gallardo, president of the Junta Directiva del Desagüe, read a speech during the inauguration in which he expressed that the need to find a solution to the *desagüe* had existed since the time when the Aztecs dominated the valley of Mexico, and that the event that gathered them together on that day was made possible by the support and enthusiasm Porfirio Díaz had given to the enterprise. He believed that the public work would deliver the city with

> hygienic conditions through the drainage of the swamps which today infest it with their smells; beauty from the cleanliness of its streets and dwellings, and the exaltation, a natural consequence of these conditions, which will place Mexico in a distinguished place amongst the largest and most populous cities on earth.[89]

The conclusion of the public works had promoted the resurgence of the capital for the third time in its history. The first had been the Aztec city, the second the colonial city, and the third the modern city. The resurgence of the city was to be accompanied by health-giving elements that would allow the country to enter into a path of future prosperity and fortune.[90]

The construction of such colossal public works could find an equivalent only in Italy. The analogy with Italy, with Rome, meant that the public works were portrayed as civilizing agents with imperial connotations. The Aztecs had not been capable of solving the problem, and neither had the Spaniards or the national government throughout most of the nineteenth century. Only Porfirio Díaz's achievements had made possible the peace and progress required for such a task, and the renewal of the capital would transform the city above ground as well as below (see Figure 8).

Other important icons of progress, such as telegraphs, ports and harbours, could also been seen throughout the country; most notable were the railroads, which extended their tracks and reached sites which had been abandoned by history and by progress. As Porfirio Díaz remarked on one occasion:

> The whistle of the train in the deserts where previously only the shriek of the savage was heard, is a sign of peace and prosperity for this noble nation, which aspires with justice to participate in the wealth that freedom and science have bestowed on the civilized world.[91]

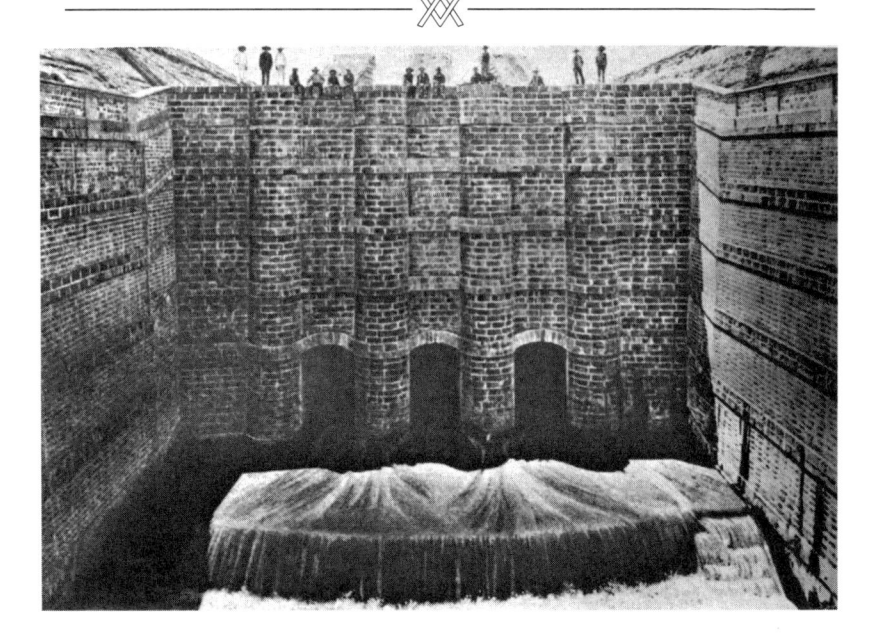

Figure 8. The Tunnel of Tequixquiac, 1900.
© Archivo Histórico del Agua, Mexico. Photograph by Alex Larrondo.

And indeed, the railroads extended throughout the country. By 1880, there were 1,073 kilometres of rail tracks; in 1884, 5,731 kilometres; in 1890, 9,544, and by 1898, the total had increased to 12,081 kilometres.[92]

But nothing could compare to the drainage works. Because of the climate of social order and peace prevalent in the nation, it had been possible to accomplish what science had deemed impossible — the control of water. Through work and perseverance, and aided by technology, the nation had been able to vanquish something that was disagreeable and a threat to public health. Shortly after the inauguration that brought together a minority of the urban population, a monument in the main plaza of Zumpango was proposed. Zumpango was the town where the administrative offices of the Dirección de las Obras del Desagüe and warehouses for the construction of the drainage system had been located. The project was defined as an artistic monument dedicated to the remembrance of the date on which the drainage system had been inaugurated.[93] In addition, on 22 March 1900, a museum was opened on the ground floor of one of the buildings occupied by la Dirección de las Obras del Desagüe del Valle de Mexico, displaying all the archaeological remains found during the construction of the Gran Canal.[94]

The construction of the monument and the museum followed the public visits to the *desagüe* that began after its inauguration. The inhabitants of the city were offered public tours. Some were advertised as outdoor excursions that promoted the idea of recreation, fresh air and healthy activity, while others had a clear educational purpose. For instance, on 1 April 1900, sixty medical students went to the drainage works, accompanied by the Professor of Hygiene, doctor Angel Gaviño.[95] In 1904, the excursions continued, as *El Imparcial* notified its readers on 15 October, stating that the enthusiasm among the families was becoming more notorious during the visits to the drainage works.[96] It was just as important to see the drainage works as it was to see the monuments placed along the Paseo de la Reforma, since they all pointed to the modernity of the city and to the climate of order and peace prevalent in the country.

The excursions to the *desagüe* were also important because they enabled all those wishing to be see them to do so in their leisure time, as a recreational activity. Leisure time became increasingly organized, whether through sports or excursions arranged by schools, clubs, workers' organizations, or by families who would enjoy the day and see with their own eyes the monumental public works that — it was hoped — would bring so many benefits to the city. The organization of recreational activities was also intended to prevent people from engaging in unhealthy or immoral activities conducive to vice, such as gambling and blood sports, in particular cockfights and bullfights.

Descriptions of other cities during the Porfiriato make it clear that programs to upgrade their sanitary conditions were also implemented, and although research has yet to be done "to examine the extent to which Mexico's provincial capitals replicated in miniature the institutional and ideological blueprint for modernization that Díaz's advisors had designed with the national metropolis in mind,"[97] some recent studies of these cities have been undertaken. In 1887, the measures taken to prevent the city of Puebla from being invaded by cholera were very much the same as those applied in the capital: the cleansing of sewers and all sites of accumulation of human and animal waste. In 1888, the city was described by Samuel Morales Pereira and Secundino Sosa, in their book *Puebla, su higiene, sus enfermedades*, as a place whose streets had no pavements, and which during the rainy season was transformed into swamps and marshes. The authors argued that the state of health or disease prevalent in a given locality was linked to environmental conditions, such as land and atmosphere; to food and drink, and in particular to the availability of water, as in the capital.[98] Panic seized Puebla in 1890 following an influenza epidemic which threatened to sweep across the city, and again the measures advised by public health officials to prevent it from spreading relied upon enhancing public hygiene. These included avoiding the stagnation of tainted water, the construction of public works, and the cultivation of cleanliness, both public and private.[99]

In 1896, the incidence of typhus among the population of Puebla was described as alarming, and the recommendations made to prevent further contagion stated that all inhabitants of the city, regardless of their social status, had to adopt and practice hygienic measures. In 1901, engineer Eduardo Bello Pérez presented the Municipal Council with a detailed sanitation project whose dictum was "Sanitation, Beauty and Utility."[100] During the last Porfirian administration of the city of Puebla (1907–11), the Municipal Council introduced a number of improvements aimed at providing better urban services, among them pavements, sewers and electricity, and by 1910, the President of the Municipal Council, Mr. Francisco de Velasco, stated that all the public works, in particular those of the Central District, were almost complete.[101]

In the south of the country, in Yucatán, Mérida was also swept by the fever of sanitary reform and by attempts to improve the city, in particular during the long tenure of Olegario Molina as governor of the state (1902–09). However, it is important to mention that before Olegario Molina's administration, the city of Mérida had been frequently swept by epidemic diseases, such as cholera in 1859, and notably by a measles epidemic in 1882–83, which took place at the same time as the henequen boom.[102] The measles epidemic occurred at a time when migrants, such as Maya villagers, Spaniards, Cubans and people from Campeche and Sonora, were attracted to the state in search of work as labour-intensive practices increased. In 1882, many of Mérida's inhabitants fled in panic to the coast and to the countryside in a desperate attempt to avoid becoming victims. But sanitary conditions in the city were so bad that many of the deaths attributed to measles were actually caused by other diseases that thrive in unsanitary and overcrowded conditions, such as tuberculosis and dysentery.[103] The streets of Mérida were described as "saharas of ill-smelling dust … in the dry season, and sloughs of despond in the wet."[104] During Olegario Molina's administration, sanitary conditions in Mérida improved, and most areas of urban life were affected: "housing, transportation, communication, public health and sanitation, education, the arts, the business community, and the urban landscape itself."[105] Molina's greatest accomplishment as a modernizer was the paving and draining of Mérida's streets, "and the city could proudly hold the name of 'White City', being clean, well lit and paved with asphalt."[106] The transformation of the city's appearance led John Kenneth Turner to state, in 1910, that "Mérida is probably the cleanest and most beautiful city in all of Mexico. It might even challenge comparison in its white prettiness with any other in the world."[107]

Hygiene in the Centennial Celebrations and the Porfirian Inheritance

Throughout the month of September and until 6 October 1910, Mexico City hosted the Centennial Celebrations of Mexico's Independence. The festivities, which coincided with Porfirio Díaz's eighth term as President and with his eightieth birthday, had a dual purpose: to create an image of national stability before an international audience; and to encourage foreign investors and visitors. Representatives from thirty-one civilized countries attended the festivities, according to the detailed information given by Genaro García in the *Crónica Oficial de las Fiestas del Primer Centenario,* and, together with the international and national guests and the inhabitants of the capital, they witnessed the inauguration of completed monuments, the inauguration of completed or improved public buildings, hospitals and a mental asylum, as well as the laying of cornerstones for new monuments, statues and buildings. Balls, banquets, international and national congresses and expositions were also organized, and parades filled the streets of the capital with a display of Mexico's history.

The efforts of the Porfirian administration in the sphere of hygiene and public health featured prominently in the festivities and were the subject of exhibitions, conferences and inaugurations. For instance, the inauguration of two public works displayed the achievements of Mexican engineering and technology and the capacity of man to tame nature for the benefit of public health, hygiene and sanitation. The water supply works would enable the city to possess abundant pure water and to demonstrate that Mexican engineers were capable of providing a solution to the most difficult scientific problems, even when they entailed obstacles that seemed insurmountable.[108] And, of course, there was the drainage system, which had its second inauguration on 26 September. Between 1900 and 1910, work on the drainage system continued, and the improvements in the Gran Canal were admired by foreigners and nationals alike.[109] Not only did the display of the *desagüe* lead to its becoming the destination of foreign visitors on train excursions, but its re-inauguration responded to the desire to show off the culmination of a secular struggle finally won during the Porfirio Díaz regime.

Among the most visited attractions was the Popular Hygiene Exhibition organized by the Superior Sanitation Council, which attracted more than 101,000 people throughout the celebrations.[110] Given the prestige enjoyed by the International Conferences on Hygiene from 1852 to 1908, gathering the most committed and renowned public health experts in cities such as London (1884), Vienna (1887), Berlin (1888), Paris (1889) and Budapest (1894), Mexico decided to host its own Hygiene Exhibition. With this exhibition, the Porfirian regime synthesized its achievements in urban improvement, made manifest the importance of a clean, ordered and hygienic city and citizenry for the modernity of the nation, and attempted to make as widely accessible as possible the basic rules of hygiene. Its primary role was to educate all its visitors.[111]

The Popular Hygiene Exhibition was opened by Dr. Eduardo Liceaga, President of the Superior Sanitation Council, on 2 September in the spacious rooms of No. 75 Avenida de Hombres Ilustres. Through statistical and graphical information relating to hygiene and sanitation, the exhibition emphasized the progress achieved between 1810 and 1910. Illustrations, maps, photographs, lantern slides and more than sixty-six models built for the exhibition showed the improvements in drinking water and sanitation, baths and toilets, housing, factories, hospitals, disinfection and school hygiene, among other things. More than 5,500 school children attended the exhibition, and more than two thousand catalogues were distributed to the public. Also prominently displayed in the exhibition were the architectural models of the new places of confinement, such as the City Jail, the General Hospital and the mental asylum, La Castañeda. To complement the exhibition, thirteen plenary lectures were given throughout the month of September by the most committed and recognized engineers, hygienists and public health officials of the time, such as Drs. Luis E. Ruiz and Domingo Orvañanos, and engineers Miguel Angel de Quevedo and Roberto Gayol.[112] And to seal the event, the book *La salubridad e higiene pública en los Estados Unidos Mexicanos* was published to commemorate the 1910 celebrations.[113]

The inaugural speech, *Progresos alcanzados en la higiene de 1810 a la fecha*, was given by Eduardo Liceaga on 2 September. In his opening remarks, he thanked the Ministry of the Interior for making possible the organization of the Exhibition of Hygiene, and made clear that the Superior Sanitation Council had to take advantage of the historic moment they were witnessing and make known the progress achieved up to that point.[114] According to Liceaga, the main concern of the Superior Sanitation Council was to spread the principles of hygiene as widely as possible, so that future generations would be healthy and vigorous, fit for work and for the advancement of civilization, be it through agriculture, industry, commerce, the arts and/or science.[115]

At this point it is important to note that by 1910, cleanliness, fresh air and pure water were regarded as essential for public health and for the progress of the nation, and that the vague concept of miasmas had gradually been replaced by that of microscopic pathogenic organisms. The emergence of bacteriology and the advances in chemistry made between the 1860s and 1890s had led to the identification of specific pathogenic organisms which caused specific diseases and to the knowledge that some diseases could be transmitted either by healthy human carriers or by animal vectors (mosquitoes, water fleas, and dog lice, among others).[116] Thus, the miasmatic theory which stressed that diseases arose from effluvia produced by decaying organic matter became an increasingly untenable one. Furthermore, the bacteriological revolution strengthened the position of the medical profession, and the hygienists — the legislators of health — publicized the new discoveries. Before these discoveries, everything had to be taken into account to prevent public health crises: overcrowding, smells, dirt, refuse and stagnant water. After the discoveries, everything still had to be taken into account, but only as it was affected by the microbe's activity, as the invisible was made visible. This shift in hygienic precepts was explicitly described by Liceaga at the conference, but this did not mean that the general public or that the scientific community at large accepted the new discoveries or that they no longer believed in the noxious effect of miasmas. The process by which the germ theory of disease gradually altered public health measures in Mexico, how the new information was transmitted and how it became accepted or assimilated are issues that this book will not explore. However, Liceaga's 1910 lecture points towards this change, and I will comment upon it very briefly.

According to Liceaga, it was impossible to describe in a single lecture all the advances hygiene had attained between 1810 and 1910. Therefore, he decided to introduce the topics that would be commented on in subsequent lectures: water provision and disposal; animal and human waste disposal; public markets; hospitals; cemeteries; prevention of disease; and the rules of public and private hygiene. The way in which he organized the information presented and the words used continually stressed the "backwardness" of previous times and the "progress" of his time: the advances in science had been linear, that is, the latest system always surpassed the previous one, and the highest point of advancement was the moment he and his contemporaries were living.[117] Liceaga believed that the unsanitary conditions in the city that for so many years had caused fear among the urban population were a thing of the past, and that most homes, industries and buildings benefited from the new system. However, he failed to give figures or be more precise, perhaps because the situation he described was far from being as efficient as he wanted the public to believe.

With regard to cholera and typhoid, he argued that it was absolutely necessary for the water consumed by humans to be pure and free of germs and bacteria and that those diseases were generally the result of carelessness of those who did not drink pure water. However, pure drinking water was limited to specific areas of the city, and most inhabitants had to resort to water drawn from wells that was unsuitable for human consumption.[118] According to Antonio Peñafiel, in 1884, the population of the city was about three hundred thousand, and water consumption was only 62.5 litres of water per head per day, a figure regarded by physicians and hygienists as unsanitary and insufficient. In 1914, a thorough study of drinking water availability written by engineer Manuel Marroquín y Rivera established that in 1899, drinking water had been not only insufficient but that its purity had been questionable, and added that by 1914, the number of houses in the capital that received drinking water did not even reach eleven thousand.[119]

Therefore, it is not surprising to find in Liceaga's conference reference to the sources of tainted water and of the water purification methods he believed would preserve the health of the urban population. During his lecture, he resorted to the use of lantern slides in order to illustrate how to preserve one's health. Lantern slides, he believed, constituted the most efficient method for educating the people and for showing them how they could filter and obtain pure water. The use of lantern slides and photography was also important in this educational mission because they portrayed "the extraordinary activity that germs possess and the prodigious velocity in which they reproduce."[120] Finally, Liceaga's conclusion was that the single most important hygienic measure was cleanliness.[121]

Cleanliness and hygienic education became more urgent following the identification of microbes and bacteria, and one of the books that analyzed in great detail the importance of the hygienic education of the Mexican people was *Higiene popular*, written by Dr. Máximo Silva during the 1890s and published in 1917.[122] According to Silva, it was imperative to bring about through education a thorough change in popular behaviour, an issue that had been on the government's agenda since the late eighteenth century.

After Porfirio Díaz's resignation and exile from the country (25 May 1911), the concern regarding the health of the city and the hygienic practices of the urban population continued. On 13 June 1911, during the interim presidency of Francisco León de la Barra (26 May–6 November 1911), a letter addressed to the Ministry of the Interior was sent by Mr. Bustamante, undersigned by twenty-five residents of the *colonias* Morelos and La Bolsa. They argued that the unsanitary conditions faced in this area of the city were a threat to their health, and that the fact that the majority of the people who lived there were poor and not accustomed to hygienic practices increased the risks to their health. They urged the government to invest resources in this area of the city, to build sewers and drainage, and explicitly criticized the Díaz administration for having spent vast amounts of money in "superfluous and luxurious public works."[123]

During both the Maderista phase of the Revolution (1910–13) and from 1913 to 1920 (the Carrancista phase), hygiene, like education, became one of the pillars upon which the revolutionary state was to stand. However, the "revolutionary image of popular vice was surprisingly consistent" with that of the

Porfiriato, as "reformers inveighed against drink, blood sports, gambling, dirt and disease."[124] In 1912, the inhabitants of the capital were subject to a fifty-cent fine if seen not wearing trousers, a measure that *El Imparcial* described as adequate if what was sought was the moral education of the popular classes.[125] In 1915, public and free bath houses were established in the capital when the city was swept by a typhus epidemic, and Venustiano Carranza allowed the Superior Sanitation Council to arrest all unclean people found in the city in order to wash them and cut their hair. Churches were only allowed to open for one hour on weekdays and two on Sundays because filthy churches were a threat to public health at times of epidemics.[126] And in December 1915, the Ministry of the Interior made public a decree issued by the executive power which outlined the measures that had to be followed in the capital to prevent the spread of the typhus epidemic:

> A special sanitary policy has been established; it is forbidden to sell pulque in small amounts; the retail sale of any kind of alcoholic drink is forbidden; public meeting places must close at 11.00 pm; dances, bazaars, soirées and meetings are forbidden; the meetings called 'wakes' are prohibited; it is forbidden that there should be pigeons, hens, dogs or animals in the houses; access to public places is prohibited to people from any social class who by their notorious dirtiness could carry on their body or clothes parasitic animals which are transmittable.[127]

Towards the end of 1917, ninety thousand people were bathed and their hair cropped in Mexico City alone,[128] and clearly, prohibiting the sale of alcoholic beverages and restricting the use of the public space to well-dressed and clean people was intimately linked to the fear of urban disorder and social upheavals in the climate of violence that was present in most of the country.

Moreover, as of 1917, the authority of the medical profession was strengthened by the deliberate attempt to reconstruct the nation, by the gradual acceptance of the germ theory of disease — which led to the gradual abandoning of the vague and catch-all concept of miasma — and the pinpointing, isolation and examination (under the microscope and in the laboratory) of the causative agents of disease. All the major issues tackled by public health officials during the Porfiriato, such as overcrowding, smells, refuse and dirt, continued to be dealt with and became increasingly associated with the previously invisible action and presence of microbes, germs and bacteria. Bacteriology made long-term plans for the sanitation of the urban environment imperative. Laboratories made microbes visible; public health officials translated the data from laboratories into the precepts of hygiene, and the public authorities legislated according to the advice given by the specialized laboratories and by the informed and competent physicians and hygienists.[129]

For the revolutionary state, all problems of hygiene and sanitation became issues directly linked with the reconstruction of the nation: a vigorous, sober, moral, industrious and healthy citizenry was required for the new social and political order. Therefore, the state had to have a more direct and comprehensive involvement, and the people had to be taught the principles of hygiene. The bacteriological discoveries of the late nineteenth century and early twentieth century proved that poor health, premature death and disease could be efficiently combatted. During the Porfiriato, many of the activities aimed at reducing the incidence of premature death and disease in Mexico City underlined the role that sanitary science would have in the achievement of this aim. The emphasis placed on the environmental aspects of the city was vital, and the control of water was regarded as one of the key elements conducive to health. After the Porfiriato, basic urban infrastructure was still considered as an element that had to be expanded as much as possible, but gradually, more attention was placed on the need to upgrade the living and working conditions, nourishment and hygienic education of the urban population. This meant that the emphasis of health policies gradually shifted from guarding municipal cleanliness to identifying human carriers and personal and domestic hygiene, regardless of the fact that the popular association of dirt and disease lingered.

The argument that the Revolution had to pursue a permanent and direct involvement in solving public health related problems can be seen in the 1916 book *La higiene en México*.[130] This book was written by engineer, economist and politician Alberto J. Pani, who was commissioned by Venustiano Carranza to carry out a detailed analysis of sanitary conditions in the capital and propose a sanitary policy for the new nation. This study was the first "Revolutionary" assessment of the sanitary conditions that had prevailed in Mexico City between 1895 and 1903, and in particular between 1904 and 1912, thus including the initial phase of the Revolution led by Francisco Madero (1910–13). The author decided to concentrate his study on the capital city because it had the largest number of people. It also had the most physicians and public health facilities, and the Superior Sanitation Council had gathered extensive statistical information to which the author had access. Pani also decided to focus on the capital because Venustiano Carranza aimed to maintain Mexico City as the "vibrant center of the nation," and to "control the city by improving its services." By May 1916, repairs on the city's parks, gardens and walks had begun, and "city planners planted trees throughout the federal district in order to beautify it, and to prevent dust storms."[131]

Pani depicted the unsanitary conditions that prevailed in the capital so that the reader could then deduce what the situation was like in other cities and towns of the republic, and action could thus be taken. The armed phase of the Revolution had critically affected the state of health of the inhabitants of the capital, and this had been aggravated by the fact that many rural dwellers had fled to the capital in search of a safe haven. Thus, many urban dwellers lacked employment and lived in overcrowded conditions, hunger was rampant and epidemic diseases, such as the typhus epidemic of 1915–16, were difficult to contain. One of the objectives of the book *La higiene en México* was to unveil the underlying causes of disease and premature death and to make that knowledge a tool for the state and for educational establishments.

According to Pani, the Superior Sanitation Council, its sanitary inspectors and the governor of the Federal District during the Porfiriato had all proved unable to offer a solution to its unsanitary conditions, regardless of the fact that since antiquity the need for the government to intervene in public health had been acknowledged. His assessment contributed to the forging of one of the predominant ideas of Mexico's historiography: that little had been accomplished during the "forced Porfirian peace." For Pani, one of the indicators that showed the degree of civilization reached by a nation was the level of advancement reached by its sanitary administration (a thesis that was also shared by his Porfirian predecessors),[132] and Mexico City's incidence of premature death reflected the backwardness of the nation. According to Pani, the death rate in the capital (42.3 per thousand) was higher than in any comparable city in the United States (16.1); it surpassed not only those of the major European cities (17.53), but also those of some Asian (Madras, 39.51) and African (Cairo, 40.15) cities.[133]

Pani summarized his main recommendations under the following headings: (i) the efficient organization of a sanitary administration for the entire Republic; (ii) obligatory sanitation for all cities with a death rate higher than the maximum limit allowed; and (iii) the raising of the moral, intellectual and economic standards of the popular sectors of society. He also believed that the revolutionary state had to take the leading role in the promotion of good health and in the prevention of premature death and disease. To this end, the diffusion of the principles and precepts of public and private hygiene was the most important task that the state had to assume. To do so, it had to rely on education and legislation.[134]

With regard to the environmental threats that were so widely discussed and analyzed during the Porfiriato, Pani argued that although the environment could exacerbate the propagation of disease — in particular of epidemics — it was known that the environment could not cause them.[135] He acknowledged that even though sanitary science was almost omnipotent, the Porfirian regime had been unable to accomplish everything it could have done to effectively drain the valley and city of Mexico, in spite of the huge amount of capital allocated to the drainage works.

He also believed that it was vital to complete the urbanization of the city, but that raising the moral, intellectual and economic standards of the Mexican people was even more urgent. The urban population suffered from a state of "physiological misery" and from "bad habits and ignorance,"[136] and the origin of this could be found in two variables: the physical environment and the moral environment. The physical environment had to be sanitized, and the moral environment transformed through education, better living and working conditions and hygiene. The urban population was also a victim of what he called "social diseases": hunger, infant mortality, tuberculosis, pneumonia, mental illness and criminality. Infant mortality was a serious problem: more than 8,100 children under the age of five died every year. The causes were poor diet, unhealthy housing, the transmission of contagious disease, and the problem was further aggravated by the lack of maternal care and education, which he described as being a moral issue. Tuberculosis and pneumonia were also huge threats to society, and caused more than

1,500 deaths each year.[137] Criminality and mental diseases were also defined as social diseases leading to a weak, diseased and unhealthy urban population, and the revolutionary state had to transform the urban and national population. Education was seen as the most suitable prescription, but Pani also acknowledged that the underlying causes of the diseased condition of the nation were the privileges and benefits that the upper classes ("los de arriba") had enjoyed throughout the history of the nation and which clearly contrasted with those of the lower classes ("los de abajo"):

> Anyone who has the slightest knowledge of our history and who can calmly survey the long and complicated process of our nation-formation, from the period before Cortés — through conquest, the Viceroyalty, the independence struggles, the upheavals, only interrupted by the forced peace of the Porfiriato, of almost a century of autonomous life — until the present age, will discover in the most outstanding manifestations of the nation's life, the unequivocal symptoms of a serious pathological state, engendered by two main causes: the sickening corruption of the upper classes and the destitution of the lower classes.[138]

Pani believed that was what required was to end the social inequalities prevalent in Mexican society. The state had to provide shelter, affordable food, education and basic urban infrastructure for all Mexicans. The goal was to promote the moral and physical hygiene of the population and to search for the means to ameliorate the living conditions of the working classes.[139] Pani extended the notion of public health to the idea of social justice, and this notion of public health was enshrined in the 1917 Constitution. Social justice, education and state intervention became crucial factors in the reconstruction of a country that was "ravaged by disease and plagued with economic problems."[140]

A key factor of this reconstruction was public health. The 1917 Constitution, through articles 1, 73 and 123, established that all Mexicans had the right to physical and mental health. The Superior Sanitation Council was transformed into the Consejo de Salubridad General. It ceased to depend on the Ministry of the Interior and was placed under the orders of the president of the Republic. In addition, a Departamento de Salubridad with federal jurisdiction was created, and its first director — doctor and general José María Rodríguez — asserted in 1918 that a "sanitary dictatorship" was an essential and unavoidable requirement for all civilized nations.[141] During the 1920s, public health and education received much attention. The Oficina de Educación Higiénica (1922) and the Escuela de Salubridad Pública (1925) were created. In 1926, a new Sanitary Code was issued, and underlined the importance that education had for the propagation of hygienic practices among the rural and urban populations. By 1927, the sanitary authorities carried out an intense hygienic campaign in schools, markets, parks and labour unions, and organized special conferences for families, mothers, wives and women in general.[142] Public health and the right of all citizens to mental and physical health became goals wherein social justice, medical research and education converged.

Public health became, during the course of the late nineteenth and early twentieth centuries, an important instrument for expanding the authority of the state, for reconciling the growing middle class and for enlarging a technically proficient state apparatus. The medical profession and new medical technology were lauded and indeed, in the paintings of the leading revolutionary artist Diego Rivera, celebrated.[143]

Epilogue

This study has explored the convergence between the rise of the discourse of public health and the development of technological and scientific solutions to sanitary problems in Mexico City during the Porfiriato. The capital city — it was argued at the time — had to display the modernization of the country, and a key feature for this display was the creation of a hygienic city that would serve as a model to the rest of the country and give confidence to foreign investors. Two factors were of crucial importance to the Porfirian modernizing project: the control of the physical environment through the construction of "the pyramids and cathedrals of the modern age,"[1] that is, public works, and the inculcation of hygienic practices among an expanding urban population.

By continually publicizing the numerous benefits that would result from the drainage system — a struggle that by the late nineteenth century had a history as long as that of the city — public health officials, sanitary engineers and state agencies avoided confronting the social inequalities that prevailed in Mexico City and greatly contributed to the high incidence of disease and premature death. Although the correlation between social inequalities and disease is confirmed in recent studies undertaken in Mexico,[2] during the final decades of the nineteenth century, the emphasis was placed on devising and applying technological, educational and scientific solutions to questions of public health. This policy served a dual purpose: to cast a veil over the social contradictions of the Porfirian modernizing project and to give a neutral foundation to their exclusionary modernization project. Through the drainage system, it was possible to make visible and tangible what no other government had managed to accomplish: that the complete control of the environment would prove that the narrative of progress had been fulfilled.

Another factor that served to emphasize the benefits that would accrue to public health from public works was the idea that unsanitary environments — plagued with miasmas — led to disease. The environmental theory of disease causation, although challenged, overshadowed and gradually discredited by the germ theory, was crucial to the assumption that the causes of the diseased condition of the city resided in the environment and in the lack of cleanliness and hygienic practices of its inhabitants. Therefore, urban sanitation and rigorous forms of cleanliness were essential for disease prevention. Only the construction of public works — and in particular the drainage system — would transform the city into a modern and hygienic urban space. And the urban population, through education, would become a law-abiding, healthy, industrious and ordered citizenry. Therefore, it was imperative to teach and make as widely accessible as possible the principles of hygiene: to bathe, dress properly, and to learn that each activity within the city had a designated space. No longer should the urban population walk the city's streets unless fully dressed; throw litter and waste wherever they found more convenient; keep domestic animals or sell fruit and vegetables in places other that those stipulated for this purpose. Thus, issues formulated as questions of public health easily became issues of public order and morality.

This overlapping of morality, public health and urban order was best portrayed in the detailed diagnosis of the city carried out by the sanitary inspectors of the Superior Sanitation Council. These thorough studies attempted to identify and isolate all elements detrimental to health, and the enforcement of the 1891 Sanitary Code provided a detailed framework of what was and was not permissible in the city.

This study has also stressed that the speculative expansion of the city led to the creation of what were perceived as being two different cities. One was defined as Ancient Mexico, or as the unsanitary city, and was located to the east and southeast of the city's centre. Its lack of the most basic urban infrastructure, its proximity to Lake Texcoco — the cesspool of the city — and the fact that it was primarily inhabited by the poorest sectors of the capital's population sharply contrasted with what became defined as Modern Mexico. The modern city was located in the *colonias* built to the southwest and west. These residential areas were built upon land that was drier and more stable, and gradually acquired sewers, paved streets, drinking water and electricity, elements defined as being palpable manifestations of the modernization of the country. It was precisely within the sanitized and modern city that the Porfirian regime displayed an official and linear version of national history, the Paseo de la Reforma becoming the axis of the hygienic city. The monuments selected and unveiled by the government presented a succession of key historical figures and events and reinforced the Porfirian regime belief that their era was one of social peace and economic progress.

Long before the late nineteenth century, the unsanitary conditions of the city and the recurrent floods had led to the elaboration of projects and proposals that aimed to modify these situations. During the late colonial period, a heightened sensitivity to foul odours and sites of accumulation and putrefaction emerged. These features of the urban environment were regarded as detrimental not only to the idea of good government or *policía*, but also to health. The Viceroy had to ensure the prosperity of New Spain so that Spain could regain its former prosperity, and a fundamental aspect of Viceroy Revillagigedo's policies was the attempt to reorganize the city and to improve its sanitary conditions. To clean up the environment and to transform the image of the city was not only a response to the impact that epidemic diseases had on society; it also became a crucial factor for the reorganization of public space. The city had traditionally been a site where multiple activities were performed side by side. However, the Bourbon authorities maintained that all activities had to take place in specifically designated sites and be performed to ensure the benefit and security of all. Baltasar Ladrón de Guevara and Hipólito Villarroel left detailed descriptions of the problems they perceived within the city and proposed measures for the good order and administration of New Spain. For Viceroy Revillagigedo, public health or sanitation became a fundamental component for the discourse of the ordered and disciplined late colonial city.

The century that separated Revillagigedo's policies from those of general Porfirio Díaz radically changed the country. Mexico's

Independence from Spain and the attempt of the emerging nation to reorganize itself was a slow and tortuous process, and Mexico City did not regain its primacy until the last third of the nineteenth century, when political authority and economic decision-making were once again centred in capital. The Porfirian monuments, together with civic improvements, public works and exhibitions, displayed an edited version of Mexico's process of modernization. The post-revolutionary governments — claiming to represent a new epoch — addressed the inequalities prevalent in Mexican society.[3] However, rather than introducing any radical change into the health policies of the Porfiriato, they continued to retain them as a basis. Thus, by 1917, the Porfirian dictum "order and progress" was supplemented by *reconstruction,* the watchword of the new regime.[4] A crucial factor in the *reconstruction* of the country was public health. The 1917 Constitution, through articles 1, 73 and 123, established that all Mexicans had the right to physical and mental health. Public health became an issue of social justice, and medical research, education, and better living and working conditions were defined as crucial for the healthy and vigorous population required by the post-revolutionary governments.

This book has left a number of issues unexplored which constitute possible lines of further inquiry. With regard to the drainage system, the following questions require an answer: What criticisms did its construction receive during the Porfiriato? Which alternative projects were proposed? What further work was carried out on the drainage system during the twentieth century and what efficiency did it have? With regard to the transition from the environmentalist theory of disease causation to the germ theory of disease, some issues that ought to be addressed include: How did the germ theory of disease become accepted by the medical and scientific community from the 1890s onwards? What was its impact in public health and sanitation policies during the 1920s and 1930s? Why were religious and military metaphors continually repeated when making reference to hygienic "campaigns," sanitary "brigades," and health "missions"? The various lines of investigation that this book has opened would benefit enormously from an interdisciplinary and regional approach to questions of public health, because after all, public health is still one of the country's most urgent requirements.

Notes

Notes to Chapter 1

1. Archivo Histórico de la Ciudad de México (hereafter AHCM), Historia, Monumentos, vol. 2276, exp. 16.
2. Ibid.
3. Jean-Antoine-Nicolas de Caritat, Marquis de Condorcet, *Esquisse d'un tableau historique des progrès de l'esprit humain,* Introduction et notes par Monique et Fran ois Hincker (Paris: Editions Sociales, 1966).
4. See Alejandra Moreno Toscano, "La constitución del espacio urbano," in *Ciudad de México: Ensayo de construcción de una historia*, edited by Alejandra Moreno Toscano (Mexico City: Instituto Nacional de Antropología e Historia – Seminario de Historia Urbana, Colección Científica 61, 1978), 167; Sonia Lombardo de Ruiz, "Ideas y proyectos urbanísticos de la ciudad de México, 1788–1850," in Moreno Toscano, *Ciudad de México* 169–71; "Discurso sobre la policía de México, 1788," in *Reflexiones y apuntes sobre la ciudad de México (fines de la colonia)* (Mexico City: Departamento del Distrito Federal, 1984), 5–9; and Ignacio González-Polo, "La ciudad de México a fines del siglo XVIII. Disquisiciones sobre un manuscrito anónimo," *Historia Mexicana* 101 (1976): 31.
5. See David Brading, "Bourbon Spain and its American Empire," in *Colonial Spanish America*, edited by Leslie Bethell (Cambridge: Cambridge University Press, 1987), 115–32.
6. While "in the seventeenth century people sinned against the King by sinning against God, in the late eighteenth century they began to be seen as sinning against the public." See Pamela Voekel, "Peeing on the Palace: Bodily Resistance to Bourbon Reforms in Mexico City," *Journal of Historical Sociology* 5, no. 2 (1992): 183.
7. John Duffy, *The Sanitarians: A History of American Public Health* (Urbana: University of Illinois Press, 1990), 1. Also see George Rosen, *A History of Public Health*, expanded edition with a new introduction by Elizabeth Fee (Baltimore and London: Johns Hopkins University Press, 1993), 1.

8 Rosen, *History of Public Health*, 1.
9 Fernando Martínez Cortés, *De los miasmas y efluvios al descubrimiento de las bacterias patógenas: Los primeros cincuenta años del Consejo Superior de Salubridad* (Mexico City: Bristol-Myers Squibb de México, 1993), 3–10; Lourdes Márquez Morfín, *La desigualdad ante la muerte en la ciudad de México: El tifo y el cólera. (1813 y 1833)* (Mexico City: Siglo XXI, 1994), 112–25; and Marcela Dávalos, *De basura, inmundicias y movimiento o de cómo se limpiaba la ciudad de México a finales del XVIII* (Mexico City: Cienfuegos, 1989).
10 The Hippocratic Corpus was written by a variety of authors, mostly between 430 and 330 BC. See *Hippocratic Writings*, edited by G. E. R Lloyd (London: Penguin, 1983), 9–12; and Caroline Hannaway, "Environment and Miasmata," in *Companion Encyclopedia of the History of Medicine*, edited by William F. Bynum and Roy Porter (London: Routledge, 1997), 1: 292–308.
11 E. J. Browne, William F. Bynum and Roy Porter, *Dictionary of the History of Science* (London: Macmillan Press, 1983), 75.
12 It must be noted that to attempt to establish a clear-cut schematization as to when religious healing practices and magical cures were supplemented by methods qualified as 'rational' or scientific is indeed far from possible. See Roy Porter, "Religion and Medicine," in *Companion Encyclopedia of the History of Medicine*, edited by Roy Porter and William F. Bynum (London, Routledge, 1993), 2: 1449–68.
13 See Roy Porter's preface to Alain Corbin, *The Foul and the Fragrant: Odour and the French Social Imagination* (London: Picador, 1994), vi.
14 Martha Eugenia Rodríguez, *Contaminación e insalubridad en la ciudad de México en el siglo XVIII* (Mexico City, Departamento de Historia y Filosofía de la Medicina – Universidad Nacional Autónoma de México, 2000).
15 Carlo Cipolla, *Miasmas and Disease: Public Health and the Environment in the pre-industrial Age* (New Haven: Yale University Press, 1992), 1–26.
16 Corbin, *Foul and the Fragrant*, 89.
17 In Peru, the urban reforms initiated in Lima by Viceroy Francisco Gil de Taboada y Lemos (1790–1796), with the assistance and recommendations of the Peruvian doctor Hipólito Unánue, also pointed towards the importance of urban sanitation for the idea of good administration and government. See David Brading, "The City in Bourbon Spanish America: Elite and Masses," *Comparative Urban Research* 8, no. 1 (1980): 72; John Tate Lanning, *The Royal Protomedicato: The Regulation of the Medical Professions in the Spanish Empire* (Durham: Duke University Press, 1985), 358–59, and Marcos Cueto (editor), *Salud, cultura y sociedad en América Latina* (Lima: IEP – Organización Panamericana de la Salud, 1996), 14–16.
18 See Donald Cooper, *Epidemic Disease in Mexico City, 1761–1813: An Administrative, Social and Medical Study* (Institute of Latin American Studies. Austin: University of Texas Press, 1965), 185.
19 See, for instance, América Molina del Villar, *Por voluntad divina: escasez, epidemias y otras calamidades en la ciudad de México, 1700–1762* (Mexico City: CIESAS, 1996).
20 Cooper, *Epidemic Disease in Mexico City*, 30–36. Also see Tate Lanning, *The Royal Protomedicato*, in particular chap. 15, "The Government, Protomedicato and Public Health," which analyses in great detail the regulations, objectives and functioning of the Royal Medical Board in Lima and Mexico City, at 351–86.

21 Cooper, *Epidemic Disease in Mexico City*, 17, 30.
22 Ibid., 53, 59–60.
23 Ignacio González-Polo, "La ciudad de México a fines del siglo XVIII — Disquisiciones sobre un manuscrito anónimo," *Historia Mexicana* 101 (1976): 30.
24 See Jean-Pierre Clement, "El nacimiento de la higiene urbana en la América española del siglo XVIII," *Revista de Indias* 171 (1983): 77–95.
25 See *Compendio de providencias de policía de México del Segundo Conde de Revillagigedo*, versión paleográfica, introducción y notas por Ignacio González-Polo, suplemento al Boletín del Instituto de Investigaciones Bibliográficas 14 (Mexico City: Universidad Nacional Autónoma de México, 1983), 13.
26 Emmanuel Le Roy Ladurie, "De l'esthétique a la pathologie," in *Histoire de la France urbaine. La Ville Classique de la Renaissance aux Revolutions*, edited by Roger Chartier et al. (Paris: Seuil, 1981), 3: 288.
27 Ibid., 288–89.
28 Ibid., 289–93. One of Louis-Sébastien Mercier's impressions of Paris was the following: "If I am asked how anyone can stay in this filthy haunt of all the vices and all the diseases piled one on top of the other, amid an air poisoned by a thousand putrid vapors, among butchers' shops, cemeteries, hospitals, drains, streams of urine, heaps of excrement ...; If I am asked how anyone lives in this abyss, where the heavy, fetid air is so thick that it can be seen, and its atmosphere smelled, for three leagues around; air that cannot circulate ... ; I would reply that familiarity accustoms the Parisian to humid fogs, maleficent vapors, and foul-smelling ooze." Quoted in Corbin, *Foul and the Fragrant*, 54.
29 Jerôme Monnet, "¿Poesía o urbanismo? Utopías urbanas y crónicas de la ciudad de México. (Siglos XVI a XX)," *Historia Mexicana* 39, no. 3 (1990): 739.
30 Ibid., 740.
31 "Discurso sobre la policía de México," versión paleográfica, introducción y notas por Ignacio González-Polo, colección Distrito Federal 4 (Mexico City: Departamento del Distrito Federal, 1984), 14. Also see Ignacio González-Polo, "La ciudad de México a fines del siglo XVIII – Disquisiciones sobre un manuscrito anónimo," *Historia Mexicana* 101 (1976): 29–47.
32 See Francisco Sedano, *Noticias de México recogidas desde el año de 1756*, coordinadas, escritas de nuevo y puestas por orden alfabético en 1800, prólogo de Joaquín García Icazbalceta (Mexico City, 1880).
33 Voekel, "Peeing on the Palace," 186. Also see Enrique Báez Macías, "Ordenanzas para el establecimiento de alcaldes de barrio en la Nueva España; ciudades de México y de San Luis Potosí," *Boletín del Archivo General de la Nación* (enero-junio 1969): 51–81; Andrés Lira, *Comunidades indígenas frente a la ciudad de México: Tenochtitlán y Tlatelolco, sus pueblos y barrios, 1812–1919* (Mexico City: El Colegio de México – El Colegio de Michoacán, 1983), 13; and Juan Pedro Viqueira Albán, *¿Relajados o reprimidos? Diversiones públicas y vida social en la ciudad de México durante el Siglo de las Luces* (Mexico City: Fondo de Cultura Económica, 1995), 232–41.
34 Enrique Báez Macías, "Ordenanzas para el establecimiento de alcaldes de barrio en la Nueva España; ciudades de México y de San Luis Potosí," 80–81.
35 "Discurso sobre la policía de México," 55.

36 See Le Roy Ladurie, "De l'esthétique a la pathologie," 288–93, and Corbin, *Foul and the Fragrant*, 48–56.
37 "Discurso sobre la policía de México," 61–62.
38 Ibid., 11, 55.
39 Ibid., 19.
40 Corbin, *Foul and the Fragrant*, 90.
41 See Carlos Sierra, *Breve historia de la navegación en la ciudad de México* (Mexico City: Departamento del Distrito Federal, 1984), 28.
42 "Discurso sobre la policía de México," 59. See also Marcela Dávalos, "La salud, el agua y los habitantes de la ciudad de México. Fines del siglo XVIII y principios del XIX," in *La ciudad de México en la primera mitad del siglo XIX*, compiled by Regina Hernández Franyuti (Mexico City: Instituto de Investigaciones Dr. José María Luis Mora, 1994), 2: 279–302.
43 "Discurso sobre la policía de México," 39.
44 Cooper, *Epidemic Disease in Mexico City*, 13.
45 Ibid., 49.
46 Ibid., 83.
47 Hipólito Villarroel, *Enfermedades políticas que padece la capital de esta Nueva España en casi todos los cuerpos de que se compone y remedios que se le deben aplicar para su curación si se quiere que sea útil al rey y al público* (written between 1785 and 1787) (Mexico City: Colección Tlahuicole 2, Editorial Porrúa, 1982). The manuscript of *Enfermedades políticas* was first published in 1831 by the historian Carlos María de Bustamante.
48 Villarroel, *Enfermedades políticas*, 31.
49 Ibid., 29.
50 Ibid., 72.
51 The body, according to this theory, had four fluids or humours — yellow bile, blood, black bile and phlegm — and the humours had their analogues in the four elements — fire, air, earth and water — respectively. See Owsei Temkin, *The Double Face of Janus and Other Essays in the History of Medicine* (London: Johns Hopkins University Press, 1977), 423–24.
52 Villarroel, *Enfermedades políticas*, 233.
53 Ibid., 173–74.
54 Ibid., 230.
55 Between 1784 and 1787, 40,000 immigrants settled in the city, largely as a consequence of an agricultural crisis in neighboring territories: see Voekel, "Peeing on the Palace," 185.
56 Villarroel, *Enfermedades políticas*, 253–55.
57 Ibid., 184–93. See also Viqueira Albán, *¿Relajados o reprimidos?*
58 See the following sections of Villarroel's *Enfermedades políticas*, "Dictamen del autor," 161–64; "Pulquerías no deben permitirse en el modo que están," 263–67; "Vinaterías," 268–69; and "Providencias que deben tomarse," 271–72.
59 Ibid., 172.
60 Juan de Viera, "Breve compendiosa narración de la ciudad de México, corte y cabeza de toda la América septentrional (1777)," in *La ciudad de México en el siglo XVIII (1690–1780): Tres crónicas*, edited by Antonio Rubial García (Mexico City: Consejo Nacional para la Cultura y las Artes, 1990), 192–93.
61 Cooper, *Epidemic Disease in Mexico City*, 34.
62 Ibid., 197–98.
63 Ibid., 36.

64 *Instrucción reservada que el Conde de Revillagigedo, dio a su sucesor en el mando, Marqués de Branciforte, sobre el gobierno de este continente en el tiempo que fue su Virrey. Con un prontuario esacto de las materias que se tocan en ella y el retrato de su autor* (Mexico City: Agustín Guiol, 1831). In this text, divided into 1,422 paragraphs, paragraphs 244 to 352 deal directly with the administration and government of Mexico City.

65 On the Enlightenment reform of burying grounds, see Pamela Voekel. "Piety and Public Space: The Cemetery Campaign in Veracruz, 1789–1810," in *Latin American Popular Culture: An Introduction*, edited by William H. Beezley and Linda A. Curcio-Nagy (Wilmington Delaware: Scholarly Resources, 2000): 1–25.

66 *Instrucción reservada que el Conde de Revillagigedo, dio a su sucesor en el mando, Marqués de Branciforte,* paragraphs 208, 227–29, 233, 246–48, 251, 303, quoted in Cooper, *Epidemic Disease in Mexico City*, 36. Also see *Compendio de providencias*: "Animales," "Vacas de Leche" and "Perros," 19–20; "Cementerios," 23; "Contagios," 34; "Desnudez," "Indios de las Repúblicas, Vestidos," 24, and "Limpieza. No. 17. Bando sobre limpieza," "Limpieza. No. 18. Bando sobre limpieza," "Reglas de Limpieza" and "Limpieza de los Barrios," 28–29.

67 See *Compendio de providencias*; David Brading, "The City in Bourbon Spanish America: Elite and Masses," *Comparative Urban Research* 8, no. 1 (1980): 72–73; Tate Lanning, *The Royal Protomedicato*, 351–59, and Pamela Voekel, "Peeing on the Palace," 183–208.

68 Márquez Morfín, *La desigualdad ante la muerte*, 57. Also see *Compendio de providencias*, 30.

69 Marcela Dávalos, *De basura, inmundicias y movimiento o de cómo se limpiaba la ciudad de México a finales del XVIII* (Mexico City: Cienfuegos, 1989), 55.

70 Ibid., 24.

71 María de Lourdes Díaz-Trechuelo Spínola et al., "El Virrey Don Juan Vicente de Güemez Pacheco, Segundo Conde de Revillagigedo (1789–1794)," in *Virreyes de Nueva España en el reinado de Carlos IV*, dirección y estudio preliminar de José Antonio Calderón Quijano, 2 Vols. (Sevilla: Escuela de Estudios Hispanoamericanos, 1972), 1: 99–100.

72 Dávalos, *De basura, inmundicia y movimiento*, 51–74, and Díaz-Trechuelo Spínola et al., "El Virrey," 94–153.

73 Voekel, "Peeing on the Palace," 196–97.

74 On the changing concepts and scope of cleanliness, and on the eighteenth century definition of the term, see Georges Vigarello, *Le propre et le sale: L'hygiène du corps depuis le Moyen Age* (Paris: Editions Seuil, 1985).

75 Corbin, *Foul and the Fragrant*, 91.

76 Francisco de la Maza, "El urbanismo neoclásico de Ignacio Castera," *Anales del Instituto de Investigaciones Estéticas* 22 (1954): 93–101. This map, as well as other maps of the city made by Ignacio Castera, can be found in SAHOP, *500 Planos de la ciudad de México, 1325–1933* (Mexico City: Secretaría de Asentamientos Urbanos y Obras Públicas, 1982), 126–29.

77 Cooper, *Epidemic Disease in Mexico City*, 33.

78 Díaz-Trechuelo Spínola et al., "El Virrey," 357.

79 See Anne Staples, "*Policia y Buen Gobierno*: Municipal Efforts to Regulate Public Behaviour, 1821–1857," In *Rituals of Rule, Rituals of Resistance. Public Celebrations and Popular Culture in Mexico*, edited by William Beezley, Cheryl English Martin and William E. French (Wilmington: Scholarly Resources, 1994), 115–26.

80 Márquez Morfín, *La desigualdad ante la muerte*, 140.
81 See Jaime E. Rodríguez O., *El proceso de la Independencia de México* (Mexico City: Instituto de Investigaciones Dr. José María Luis Mora, 1992); Marcelo Carmagnani, "Territorios, provincias y estados: las transformaciones de los espacios políticos en México, 1750–1850," in *La fundación del Estado mexicano, 1821–1855*, coordinated by Josefina Zoraida Vázquez (Mexico City: Nueva Imagen, 1994), 39–73.
82 See Andrés Lira, "Legalización del espacio: la ciudad de México y Distrito Federal, 1874–1884," in *Construcción de la legitimidad política en México*, coordinated by Brian Connaughton, Carlos Illades and Sonia Pérez Toledo (Mexico: El Colegio de Michoacán – Universidad Autónoma Metropolitana – Universidad Nacional Autónoma de México – El Colegio de México, 1999), 323–50.
83 See "Bando de policía y buen gobierno," issued by the governor of the Federal District, José Mendivil, on 7 February 1825, reproduced in José Alvarez Amézquita et al., *Historia de la salubridad y de la asistencia en México* (Mexico City: Secretaría de Salubridad y Asistencia, 1960), 1: 205–13.
84 On the 1833 cholera epidemic and the political climate of Mexico, see Paulo Morgan Simoes de Carvalho, "*El azote que hoy nos amaga*: cholera, reaction and insurrection in Mexico, 1833" (M.A. diss., San José State University, 1996), 48–77, and Donald F. Stevens, "Temerse la ira del cielo: los conservadores y la religiosidad popular en los tiempos del cólera," in *El conservadurismo mexicano en el siglo XIX (1810–1910)*, coordinated by Humberto Morales and William Fowler (Mexico: Benemérita Universidad Autónoma de Puebla – University of Saint Andrews, 1999), 87–101. See also Charles A. Hutchinson, "El cólera de 1833: el Día del Juicio en México," *Paginas de los Trabajadores del Estado*, Mexico City (March 1984): 14–26; Miguel Angel Cuenya et al., *El cólera de 1833: una nueva patología en México: Causas y efectos* (Mexico City: Instituto Nacional de Antropología e Historia, Colección Divulgación, 1992); Márquez Morfín, *La desigualdad ante la muerte*, 280, 268–323. Also see Pilar Velasco, "La epidemia de cólera de 1833 y la mortalidad en la ciudad de México." *Estudios Demográficos y Urbanos* 19 (1992): 95–135.
85 Simoes de Carvalho, *"El azote que hoy nos amaga,"* 48–77.
86 For a detailed comparative analysis of state regulation and intervention in matters relative to public health and the medical profession during the late eighteenth century and throughout the course of the nineteenth century, see Matthew Ramsey, "The Politics of Professional Monopoly in Nineteenth-Century Medicine: The French Model and Its Rivals," in *Professions and the French State, 1700–1900*, edited by Gerald L. Geison (Philadelphia: University of Pennsylvania Press, 1984), 225–305.
87 On the cholera epidemics of the nineteenth century, see, among many other studies, Charles Rosenberg, *The Cholera Years: The United States in 1832, 1849 and 1866. With a new Afterword* (Chicago and London: The University of Chicago Press, 1987); Fran ois Delaporte, *Disease and Civilization: The Cholera in Paris* (Cambridge, MA.: MIT Press, 1986), and Richard J. Evans, *Death in Hamburg: Society and Politics in the Cholera Years, 1830–1910* (Oxford: Clarendon Press, 1987).
88 Vijay Prashad, "Native Dirt/Imperial Ordure: The Cholera of 1832 and the Morbid Resolutions of Modernity," *Journal of Historical Sociology* 7, no. 3 (1994): 243, 248, and Vigarello, *Le propre et le sale*.

89 On the nineteenth century Sanitary Conferences, see Norman Howard-Jones, *The Scientific Background of the International Sanitary Conferences, 1851–1938* (Geneva: World Health Organization, 1975). See also William F. Bynum, *Science and the Practice of Medicine in the Nineteenth Century* (Cambridge: Cambridge University Press, 1994), 142–46.

90 "Noviembre 21 de 1831. Ley – Cesación del Real Tribunal del Protomedicato y creación de una junta nombrada Facultad Médica del Distrito Federal," in Manuel Dublán and José María Lozano, *Legislación mexicana o colección completa de las disposiciones legislativas expedidas desde la Independencia de la República* (Mexico City: Imprenta de Eduardo Dublán, 1876) 2: 403–4. See also Alvarez Amézquita et al., *Historia de la salubridad*, 1: 218–28.

91 On Mexico's scientific and medical associations during the course of the nineteenth century, see Juan José Saldaña and Luz Fernanda Azuela, "De amateurs a profesionales. Las sociedades científicas mexicanas en el siglo XIX," *Quipu: Revista Latinoamericana de Historia de las Ciencias y la Tecnología* 11, no. 2 (May–August 1994): 135–72.

92 See also "Ordenanzas formadas por la Junta Departamental en el año de 1840 por el Gobernador Dr. Don Luis G. Vieyra," in particular chap. 3: "Salubridad pública." Reproduced in Alvarez Amézquita et al., *Historia de la salubridad*, 1: 236–47.

93 Alvarez Amézquita et al., *Historia de la salubridad*, 1: 250–52.

Notes to Chapter 2

1 Jean-Pierre Goubert, *The Conquest of Water: The Advent of Health in the Industrial Age* (London: Polity Press, 1986), 110.

2 See Mílada Bazant, *Historia de la educación durante el porfiriato* (Mexico City: El Colegio de México, 1993), 231–48, 262–67.

3 Charles Hale, "Political and Social Ideas," in *Latin America: Economy and Society, 1870–1930*, edited by Leslie Bethell. (Cambridge: Cambridge University Press, 1984), 241, and Charles Hale, *The Transformation of Liberalism in Late-Nineteenth Century Mexico* (Princeton, NJ: Princeton University Press, 1989), 205–44.

4 Hale, "Political and Social Ideas," 241. Positivism first entered the intellectual environment of Mexico during the 1860s with Dr. Gabino Barreda, and its main concern was the reorganization of higher education, not politics. It was not until 1878 that the formal enunciation of 'scientific politics' was presented by Justo Sierra, Francisco G. Cosmes and Telésforo García, among others, through *La Libertad* (1878–1884), a daily newspaper subsidized by the government of Porfirio Díaz.

5 Francisco G. Cosmes in *La Libertad*, 11 October 1878, quoted in Hale, *Transformation of Liberalism*, 34.

6 Some of the works that underline the utility of statistical information and that point towards the "progress" reached by the country due to the climate or order and peace that prevailed are: Antonio García Cubas, *Atlas Geográfico y estadístico de los Estados Unidos Mexicanos* (Mexico City: Oficina Tipográfica de la Secretaría de Fomento, 1884); and *Cuadro Geográfico, estadístico, descriptivo e histórico de los Estados Unidos Mexicanos* (Mexico City: Oficina Tipográfica de la Secretaría de Fomento, 1885). Railroads also

became the focal point of much statistical work: see *Reseña histórica y estadística de los ferrocarriles de jurisdicción federal desde el 1 de enero de 1895 hasta el 31 de diciembre de 1899* (Mexico City: Tipografía de la Dirección General de Telégrafos Federales, 1900). See in particular the work *Los Estados Unidos Mexicanos: Sus progresos en veinte años de paz, 1877–1897* (New York: H. A. Rost & Co., 1899).

7 María Dolores Morales, "La expansión de la ciudad de México en el siglo XIX: El caso de los fraccionamientos," in *Investigaciones sobre la historia de la ciudad de México* (Cuadernos de Trabajo del Departamento de Investigaciones Históricas, Mexico City: Instituto Nacional de Antropología e Historia, 1974), 74.

8 Moisés González Navarro, *Historia moderna de Mexico. El porfiriato. La vida social* (Mexico City: Editorial Hermes, 1957), 29.

9 See "Table 1. Población por entidades federativas. Años de 1877 a 1910," in *Estadísticas sociales del porfiriato, 1877–1910* (Mexico City: Talleres Gráficos de la Nación, 1956), 7–8. The only available information for the urban/rural breakdown of the Mexican population during the Porfiriato is the data for 1910.

10 See Agustín Reyes's report of the activities carried out by the Statistics Commission of the Superior Sanitation Council during 1879 in Alvarez Amézquita et al., *Historia de la salubridad*, 1: 291.

11 Gordon Schendel, *Medicine in Mexico: From Aztec Herbs to Betatrons* (Austin: University of Texas Press, 1968), 148. According to Dr. Peñafiel, the mortality rate in 1895 was 31 per 1,000 live births and 31.9 per 1,000 live births in 1907. In 1961, Benítez Zenteno calculated that life expectancy at birth during the Porfiriato decreased from 29.5 years in 1895 to 27.4 in 1910. See Raul Benítez Zenteno, *Analisis Demográfico de México* (Mexico City: Instituto de Investigaciones Sociales, Universidad Nacional Autónoma de México, 1961), 62.

12 Hale, *Transformation of Liberalism*, 155. Other journals devoted to the popularization of the sciences and of hygiene were the following: *Gaceta Médica de México. Organo de la Academia Nacional de Medicina* (1864–1915); *El Observador Médico: Publicación científica de la Asociación Médica 'Pedro Escobedo'* (1869–1883; 1886; 1901–1905 and 1908); *La Naturaleza. Publicación Científica de la Sociedad Mexicana de Historia Natural* (1869–1903; 1910–1911); *Boletín del Ministerio de Fomento* (1877–1886); *La Escuela de Medicina. Periódico Científico* (1879–1909; 1912; 1914); *La Moralidad. Semanario dedicado exclusivamente al mejoramiento de las costumbres y la extirpación de los vicios* (1885–1886); and *La Mujer Mexicana. Revista científico-literaria consagrada al progreso y perfeccionamiento de la mujer mexicana* (1904–1908), among others. A detailed review of the medical journals and newspapers published during the course of the nineteenth century in Mexico is found in: Martha Eugenia Rodríguez, "Semanarios, gacetas, revistas y periódicos médicos del siglo XIX mexicano," *Boletín del Instituto de Investigaciones Bibliográficas – Nueva época* 2, no. 2 (1997): 61–96.

13 González Navarro, *Historia moderna de México*, 5.

14 Alvarez Amézquita et al., *Historia de la salubridad*, 1: 279.

15 For a detailed historical analysis of the statistical movement in Mexico and its consolidation during the Porfiriato, see Sergio de la Peña and James Wilkie, *La estadística económica en México: Los orígenes* (Mexico City: Siglo XXI, 1994), 5–128, in particular 93–121.

16 González Navarro, *Historia moderna de México*, 8.
17 Antonio Peñafiel (1839–1922) studied medicine (1867), was one of the founders of the Sociedad de Historia Natural, director of the Dirección General de la Estadística, and edited numerous historical works about Ancient Mexico, among them *Monumentos del Arte Mexicano Antiguo*; *Nomenclatura Geográfica, Etimológica y Geroglífica de México* and *Teotihuacán*. See *Diccionario Porrúa de historia, biografía y geografía de México* (Mexico City: Editorial Porrúa, 1976), 1601. In 1889, Dr. Peñafiel was commissioned to the Paris Exposition Universelle, where he built the "Pabellón Azteca." On this "Pabellón Azteca," see his *Explicación del Edificio Mexicano para la Exposición Internacional de París en 1889* (Mexico City: 1889). He also wrote an exhaustive study about water availability in Mexico City: see his *Memoria sobre las Aguas Potables en México* (Mexico City: Oficina Tipográfica de la Secretaría de Fomento, 1884).
18 On the importance that medical statistics acquired in Mexico during the final decades of the nineteenth century, see Laura Cházaro García, "Medir y valorar los cuerpos de una nación: un ensayo sobre la estadística médica del siglo XIX mexicano" (Ph.D. diss., Facultad de Filosofía y Letras, Universidad Nacional Autónoma de México, 2000).
19 Luis E. Ruiz, *Tratado elemental de higiene* (Mexico City: Oficina Tipográfica de la Secretaría de Fomento, 1904), 254–55. Also see the work done by Isidro Epstein, *La mortalidad en México* (Mexico City: Sociedad Mexicana de Geografía y Estadística, 1894).
20 Ruiz, *Tratado elemental*, 496.
21 See Pablo Piccato, "'El Paso de Venus por el disco del Sol': Criminality and Alcoholism in the Late Porfiriato," *Mexican Studies/Estudios Mexicanos* 2, no. 2 (Summer 1995): 209, who argues that personal observations alongside statistics were crucial for the study of alcoholism and criminality during the Porfiriato. Proof of the lack of continuity and consistency in the Porfirian statistics can be appreciated by looking at the *Estadísticas Sociales del Porfiriato*; see in particular the "Preface" written by Moisés González Navarro, 5–6.
22 Rosen, *History of Public Health*, 235–39.
23 For a thorough analysis of the public health or sanitary movement in Great Britain, France, Germany and the United States during the course of the nineteenth century, see Rosen, *History of Public Health*, 168–269. For the United States and France, see Daniel Wilsford, *Doctors and the State: The Politics of Health Care in France and the United States* (Durham: Duke University Press, 1991); for Great Britain, see *Urban Disease and Mortality in Nineteenth-Century England*, edited by Robert Woods and John Woodward (New York: St. Martin's Press, 1984).
24 Bynum, *Science and the Practice*, 87–91. See also Dorothy Porter, "Public Health," in *Companion Encyclopedia of the History of Medicine*, edited by William F. Bynum and Roy Porter (London: Routledge, 1993), 2: 1241–50; and *The History of Public Health and the Modern State*, edited by Dorothy Porter (Amsterdam – Atlanta: Editions Rodopi, 1994).
25 Goubert, *Conquest of Water*, 103.
26 Ann F. La Berge, *Mission and Method: The Early-Nineteenth-Century French Public Health Movement* (Cambridge: Cambridge University Press, 1992), 20, 54–55. In England, the statistical movement flourished in the 1830s, when the relationship between poverty and disease was seen as crucial for

understanding the high incidence of premature death among the population. "The new science of social reform, statistics (the tool of the 'statist'; the student of the state) was used by Edwin Chadwick, who measured the incidence of disease and mortality by compiling figures from statistics and whose results were published in the *Report on the sanitary conditions of the labouring population of 1842.* See Christopher Lawrence, *Medicine in the Making of Modern Britain, 1700–1920* (London: Routledge, 1994), 43.

27 De la Peña and Wilkie, *La estadística económica*, 73–74.
28 José Güijosa, *El Valle de México: Ventajas que resultarán a la salud pública con el desagüe,* Tesis para el examen general de medicina, cirugía y obstetricia, Escuela Nacional de Medicina (Mexico City: Imprenta de Joaquín G. Campos y Comp, 1892), 27. The following specialized studies carried out during the Porfiriato point towards the growing concern about the need to control the environment: Ladislao de Belina, "Medios para mejorar la canalización de México." *Boletín de la Sociedad Mexicana de Geografía y Estadística* (Mexico City: Imprenta de Francisco Díaz de León, 1897); Francisco Bulnes, *El desagüe del Valle de México a la luz de la higiene* (Mexico City: Oficina Impresora de Estamillas, Tipografía Palacio Nacional, 1892); Florentino Sariol, *Ligera consideración acerca de la influencia nociva que ejercen las materias fecales sobre la salubridad: medidas higiénicas para combatir dicha influencia* (Mexico City: Imprenta de Francisco Díaz de León, 1887).
29 Goubert, *Conquest of Water*, 23–24.
30 Genaro Raigosa, *Discurso pronunciado por el Sr. Senador Genaro Raigosa en la sesión del 16 de noviembre de 1881 sobre el contrato celebrado entre el Secretario de Fomento y el Sr. Antonio de Mier y Celis para el desagüe y saneamiento de la ciudad y del Valle de México* (Mexico City: Imprenta del Gobierno en Palacio, 1881). The Minister of Development was at the time Carlos Pacheco, and General Manuel González held the presidency from 1 December 1880 to 30 November 1884. General Porfirio Díaz held the Ministry of Development from 1 December 1880 to 23 May 1881.
31 Raigosa, *Discurso pronunciado*, 7.
32 The valley of Mexico, it must be noted, technically is not a "valley" but a basin, for it lacks a natural outlet for the water found within it.
33 Antonio García Cubas, *Atlas geográfico y estadístico de los Estados Unidos Mexicanos* (Mexico City: Oficina Tipográfica de la Secretaría de Fomento, 1884), 11.
34 Raigosa, *Discurso pronunciado*, 15.
35 Ibid., 16.
36 Ibid., 17.
37 Ibid., 16.
38 Julio Guerrero, *La génesis del crimen en México: Estudio de psiquiatría social* (Mexico City and Paris: Librería de la Viuda de Charles Bouret, 1901), 21–22.
39 Dávalos, *De basura, inmundicias y movimiento*, 133.
40 Antonio Peñafiel, *Memoria sobre las aguas potables en México* (Mexico City: Oficina Tipográfica de la Secretaría de Fomento, 1884), 129.
41 Ibid.
42 Ibid., 31.
43 Raigosa, *Discurso pronunciado*, 9.
44 Ibid., 14.

45 Bynum, *Science and the Practice*, 59.
46 Temkin, *The Double Face*, 469.
47 Corbin, *Foul and the Fragrant*, 14–15.
48 Ibid., 10–11, and Nancy Tomes, *The Gospel of Germs: Men, Women, and the Microbe in American Life* (Cambridge, Massachusetts: Harvard University Press, 1998), 26–29.
49 Corbin, *Foul and the Fragrant*, 1.
50 Goubert, *Conquest of Water*, 60.
51 Raigosa, *Discurso pronunciado*, 12.
52 On the germ theory of disease and its gradual acceptance in the United States, see Tomes, *Gospel of Germs*, 23–48, and Margaret Pelling, "Contagion/germ theory/specificity," in *Companion Encyclopedia of the History of Medicine*, edited by William F. Bynum and Roy Porter (London: Routledge, 1993), 1: 309–34.
53 Manuel de la Fuente, *Estudio sobre las aplicaciones de la higiene contra la invasión del cólera epidémico*, Presentado en el examen de medicina y cirugía (Mexico City: Oficina Tipográfica de la Secretaría de Fomento, 1885), 9. In 1882, Robert Koch identified the bacilli that caused tuberculosis, and in 1883 the bacilli that caused cholera. See Rosen, *History of Public Health*, 290–91.
54 Miguel E. Bustamante, "La situación epidemiológica de México en el siglo XIX," in *Ensayos sobre la historia de las epidemias en México*, edited by Enrique Florescano and Elsa Malvido (Mexico City: Instituto Mexicano del Seguro Social – Colección Salud y Seguridad Social, Serie Historia, 1982), 2: 443.
55 Raigosa, *Discurso pronunciado*, 18.
56 Ibid., 30.
57 Hale, *Transformation of Liberalism*, 25–26, 147, 233.
58 *Diccionario Porrúa de historia, biografía y geografía de México*, Quinta edición, corregida y aumentada con un suplemento (Mexico City: Editorial Porrúa, 1986), 2527.
59 Ruiz, *Tratado elemental*, 3, 6.
60 Ibid., 146.
61 Ibid., 21.
62 José Alfaro, *Higiene pública: Algunas palabras acerca de la influencia higiénica de las arboledas y necesidad de reglamentar su uso entre nosotros*, Prueba escrita para el examen general de medicina, cirugía y obstetricia (Mexico City: Terrazas Impresora, San José de Gracia 5, 1892), 12–13. See also José Guadalupe Lobato, "Higiene pública. Los arbolados, los bosques montañosos y los planos, los jardines, las huertas y los sembrados en las comarcas geográficas intercontinentales," *Gaceta Médica de México* 16, no. 15 (1 August 1881): 249–59, 274–82, and Jesús Sánchez, "Higiene de los jardines públicos y particulares de la ciudad de México," *Gaceta Médica de México* 21, no. 3 (1 February 1886): 45–53, 74–78.
63 Alfaro, *Higiene pública*, 15, 31.
64 Ibid., 31.
65 Thomas M. Reese and Carol McMichael Reese, "Revolutionary Urban Legacies: Porfirio Díaz's Celebrations of the Centennial of Mexican Independence in 1910," in *Estudios de Arte y Estética 37. XVII Coloquio Internacional de Historia del Arte. Arte, Historia e Identidad en América: Visiones Comparativas* (Mexico City: Instituto de Investigaciones Estéticas

– Universidad Nacional Autónoma de México,1994) 2: 368–69. See also María Estela Eguiarte Sakar, "Los jardines en México y la idea de ciudad decimonónica." *Historias* 27. Revista de la Direcccción de Estudios Históricos del Instituto Nacional de Antropología e Historia (October 1991-March 1992): 129–38. Miguel Angel de Quevedo's urban design philosophy can be found in *Espacios libres y reservas forestales de las ciudades, su adaptación á jardines, parques y lugares de juego, su aplicación a la Ciudad de México* (Mexico City: Gomy Busón, 1911). A draft of Quevedo's *Espacios Libres*... can be found in the Archivo Histórico de la Secretaría de Salud (hereafter AHSS), Salubridad, Presidencia, Secretaría, exp. 6, caja 33.
66 Ruiz, *Tratado elemental*, 154.
67 Ibid., 153, 168, 182.
68 Ibid., 166.
69 Liceaga's statement can be found in AHCM, Consejo Superior de Gobierno del Distrito, Salubridad e higiene, vol. 645, exp. 21. See González Navarro, *Historia Moderna de México*, for Orvañanos' emphasis upon cleanliness, 43–44.
70 Mary Douglas, *Purity and Danger: An Analysis of the Concepts of Pollution and Taboo* (London: Routledge, 1994), 160–61.
71 González Navarro, *Historia Moderna de México*, 43–44.
72 Ruiz, *Tratado elemental*, 156.
73 Ibid., 450.
74 The following selection of articles published in Mexico City in *El Imparcial* during 1898 make reference to both the germ and the miasmatic theory of disease: "Higiene Doméstica," *El Imparcial*, 8 July 1898; "La higiene de las calles," *El Imparcial*, 17 July 1898; "La higiene de la piel," *El Imparcial*, 13 November 1898; "Prescripciones útiles. Las enfermedades contagiosas," *El Imparcial*, 27 December 1898. See also "Un poco sobre besos," *La mujer mexicana. Revista mensual, científico literaria* 1, no. 7 (1904): 9, and Laura M. Cuenca, "Las necesidades de México: México necesita aseo," in *La mujer mexicana. Revista mensual, científico literaria* 2, no. 4 (1905): 1–2. For an analysis of the importance that personal hygiene acquired due to the germ theory of disease in Mexico during the final decades of the nineteenth century, see Claudia Agostoni, "Las delicias de la limpieza: la higiene en la ciudad de México," in *Bienes y vivencias: El siglo XIX mexicano*, edited and compiled by Anne Staples, in *Historia de la vida cotidiana en México*, coordinated by Pilar Gonzalbo (Mexico City: El Colegio de México – Fondo de Cultura Económica, in press).
75 See Andrew McClary, "Germs are Everywhere: The Germ Threat as Seen in Magazine Articles, 1890–1920," *Journal of American Culture* 3, nos. 1–2 (1980): 33–46; Naoemi Rogers, "Germs with Legs: Flies, Disease and the New Public Health," *Bulletin of the History of Medicine* 63 (1989): 599–617, and Nancy Tomes, "The Private Side of Public Health: Sanitary Science, Domestic Hygiene, and the Germ Theory, 1870–1900," *Bulletin of the History of Medicine* 64 (1990): 509–39.
76 Donald Reid, *Sewers and Sewermen: Realities and Representations* (Cambridge Massachusetts: Harvard University Press, 1991), 18.

Notes to Chapter 3

1. AHCM, Demarcación, Cuarteles, vol. 650, exp. 29.
2. Jorge Eduardo Hardoy, "Theory and Practice of Urban Planning in Europe, 1850–1930: Its Transfer to Latin America," in *Rethinking the Latin American City*, edited by Richard M. Morse and Jorge E. Hardoy (Baltimore: Johns Hopkins University Press, 1992), 21.
3. María Dolores Morales, "La expansión de la ciudad de México en el siglo XIX: El caso de los fraccionamientos," in *Investigaciones sobre la historia de la ciudad de México,* Cuadernos de Trabajo del Departamento de Investigaciones Históricas (Mexico City: Instituto Nacional de Antropología e Historia (1974), 74.
4. Some studies on late nineteenth century and early twentieth century health care and sanitation in Latin American cities include the following: Carl Murdock, "Physicians, the State and Public Health in Chile, 1881–1891," *Journal of Latin American Studies* 27 (1995): 551–67; Sidney Chalhoub, "The Politics of Disease Control: Yellow Fever and Race in Nineteenth Century Rio de Janeiro," *Journal of Latin American Studies* 25 (1993): 441–63; Nicolau Sevcenko, *A Revolta da Vacina. Mentes insanas em corpos rebeldes* (São Paulo: Editora Scipione, 1993); Ron F. Pineo, "Misery and Death in the Pearl of the Pacific: Health Care in Guayaquil, Ecuador, 1870–1925," *Hispanic American Historical Review* 70, no. 4 (1990): 609–37; Teresa Meade, "Living Worse and Costing More: Resistance and Riot in Rio de Janeiro," *Journal of Latin American Studies* 21 (1989): 241–66; Jeffrey D. Needell, "The *Revolta Contra Vacina* of 1904: The Revolt Against 'Modernization' in *Belle-Époque* Rio de Janeiro," *Hispanic American Historical Review* 67 (1987): 233–69 and Teresa Meade, "Civilising Rio de Janeiro: The Public Health Campaign and the Riot of 1904," *Journal of Social History* 20, no. 2 (1987): 301–22, among others.
5. Christopher Abel, *Health, Hygiene and Sanitation in Latin America, c. 1870 to c. 1950* (Institute of Latin American Studies, Research Papers 42. London: University of London, 1996), 3. On criminality, policing and detection methods in Mexico City from the 1870s to the 1930s, see Robert Buffington, *Criminal and Citizen in Modern Mexico* (Lincoln: University of Nebraska Press, 1999); Pablo Piccato, *City of Suspects. Crime in Mexico City, 1900–1931* (Durham: Duke University Press, 2001); Elisa Speckman Guerra, *Crimen y castigo. Legislación penal, interpretaciones de la criminalidad y administración de justicia (Ciudad de México, 1871–1910)* (Mexico City: El Colegio de México – Universidad Nacional Autónoma de México, 2002); and Beatríz Urías Horcasitas, *Indígena y criminal. Interpretaciones del derecho y la antropología en México, 1871–1921* (Mexico City: Universidad Iberoamericana, 2000).
6. For an analysis of the impact of the expansion of Mexico City on the indigenous population, see Andrés Lira, *Comunidades indígenas frente a la ciudad de México. Tenochtitlán y Tlatelolco, sus pueblos y barrios, 1812–1919* (Mexico City: El Colegio de México – El Colegio de Michoacán, 1983), 382–85.
7. María Dolores Morales, "La expansión de la ciudad de México en el siglo XIX: El caso de los fraccionamientos," in *Ciudad de México. Ensayo de construcción de una historia,* edited by Alejandra Moreno Toscano (Mexico City: Instituto Nacional de Antropología e Historia – Seminario de Historia Urbana, Colección Científica 61, 1978), 194.

8 Ibid., 194. Also see Alejandra López Monjardín, *Hacia la ciudad capital: México, 1790–1870* (Mexico City: Dirección de Estudios Históricos – Instituto Nacional de Antropología e Historia, 1985), 83–152.
9 Morales, "La expansión de la ciudad de México en el siglo XIX" (1974), 77.
10 AHCM, Colonias, vol. 519, exp. 1.
11 Morales, "La expansión de la ciudad de México en el siglo XIX" (1974), 77.
12 Ibid., 84. Also see Jorge Jiménez Muñoz, *La traza del poder: historia de la política y los negocios urbanos en el Distrito Federal, de sus orígenes a la desaparición del ayuntamiento, 1824–1928* (Mexico City: CODEX Editores, 1993).
13 María Dolores Morales, "La expansion de la ciudad de Mexico (1858–1910)," in *Atlas de la Ciudad de México*, edited by Gustavo Garza (Mexico City: Departamento del Distrito Federal – El Colegio de México, 1987), 65.
14 María Dolores Morales, "Francisco Somera y el primer fraccionamiento de la ciudad de México," in *Formación y desarrollo de la burguesia en México*, edited by Ciro Cardoso (Mexico City: Siglo XXI, 1978a), 192. Also see AHCM, Colonias, vol. 519, exp. 23 bis: "Bases generales de trazo é higiene a que deben sujetarse las nuevas colonias"; and vol. 519, exp. 27: "Bases á que deberán sujetarse la creación de nuevas colonias en la municipalidad de México."
15 On the importance of French architecture and urban design in Mexico City, see Federico Fernández Christlieb, "La influencia francesa en el urbanismo de la ciudad de México: 1775–1910," in *México – Francia. Memoria de una sensibilidad común, siglos XVIII-XX*, compiled by Javier Pérez Siller (Mexico: Benemérita Universidad Autónoma de Puebla – El Colegio de San Luis A.C. – CEMCA, 1998), 227–65.
16 For an analysis of the urban reforms of Rio de Janeiro and the selective and pragmatic incorporation of elements of European urban design and the emphasis on creating efficient public works during the last decades of the nineteenth century, see Jaime Larry Benchimol, *Pereira Passos: Um Haussmann Tropical. A renova ão urbana da cidade do Rio de Janeiro no início do século XX* (Rio de Janeiro: Biblioteca Carioca, 1990). For Buenos Aires, see James Scobie, *Buenos Aires: Plaza to Suburb, 1870–1910* (New York: Oxford University Press, 1974), 21–32. A very useful overview of the selection and incorporation of European and North American urban models in Latin America from the 1850s to the 1930s can be found in Hardoy, "Theory and Practice of Urban Planning," 20–49.
17 Morales, "La expansión de la ciudad de México (1858–1910)," 65.
18 The impact and changes brought about by the railroads on the economy and social organization of the country during the Porfirian regime has been studied by numerous scholars, among them John H. Coatsworth, *El impacto económico de los ferrocarriles en el Porfiriato: Crecimiento contra desarrollo* (Mexico City: Ediciones Era, 1976). Also see Alejandra Moreno Toscano, "Cambios en los patrones de urbanización en México, 1810–1910," *Historia Mexicana* 22 (1972): 184.
19 Adolfo Prantl and José Groso, *La ciudad de México: Novísima guía universal de la capital de la república mexicana* (Mexico City: Juan Buxó y Compañía editores, Librería Madrileña, 1901), 688.
20 Hira de Gortari and Regina Hernández Franyuti, *Memoria y Encuentros: La Ciudad de México y el Distrito Federal (1824–1928)* (Mexico City: Instituto de Investigaciones Dr. José María Luis Mora – Departamento del Distrito Federal, 1988), 373.

21 Jesús Galindo y Villa, *Historia sumaria de la Ciudad de México*, 1925, quoted in Diego López Rosado, *Los servicios públicos de la ciudad de México* (Mexico City: Editorial Porrúa, 1976), 185, my italics.
22 See Manuel Rivera Cambas' *México pintoresco, artístico y monumental* (Mexico City: Imprenta de la Reforma, 1883), 145–46, and Guillermo Prieto, *Memoria de mis tiempos* (Mexico City: Librería de Charles Bouret, 1906).
23 Márquez Morfín, *La desigualdad ante la muerte*, 124–25.
24 Prantl and Groso, *La ciudad de México*, 421.
25 "Febrero 1 de 1886. Gobierno del Distrito. Bando sobre aseo de las vías públicas de la ciudad de México," in Dublán and Lozano, *Legislación mexicana*, 13: 364–65.
26 Prantl and Groso, *La ciudad de México*, 689.
27 See Jorge Salessi, *Médicos maleantes y maricas: Higiene, criminología y homosexualidad en la construcción de la nación Argentina. (Buenos Aires: 1871–1914)* (Buenos Aires: Estudios Culturales – Beatriz Viterbo Editora, 1995), 19–21; and Diego Armus, "Tutelaje, higiene y prevención. Una ciudad modelo para la Argentina de comienzos de siglo," in *Medio Ambiente y Urbanización: Homenaje a Jorge E. Hardoy* (Buenos Aires: Instituto Internacional del Medio Ambiente y Desarrollo, IIEDAL, 1993), 79–88.
28 William Beezley, *Judas at the Jockey Club and Other Episodes of Porfirian Mexico* (Lincoln and London: University of Nebraska Press, 1987), 9, 134.
29 *La voz de México*, 8 September 1878.
30 González Navarro, *Historia moderna de México*, 119.
31 Ibid., 120.
32 Emilio Rabasa, *El Cuarto Poder y Moneda Falsa* (Mexico City: Editorial Porrúa, 1970), 11.
33 Ibid., 12–13.
34 For a detailed analysis of the educational system and its effectiveness during the Porfiriato, see Mílada Bazant, *Historia de la educación durante el Porfiriato* (Mexico City: El Colegio de México, 1993). Also see Mary Kay Vaughan, *The State, Education and Social Class in Mexico, 1880–1928* (De Kalb: Northern Illinois University Press, 1982).
35 AHCM, Policía, Salubridad, Cólera morbus, vol. 3676, exp. 31.
36 Ibid.
37 Bazant, *Historia de la educación durante el Porfiriato*, 241, and Mílada Bazant, "La enseñanza y la práctica de la ingeniería durante el Porfiriato," *Historia Mexicana* 3 (1984): 254–97.
38 "Table 14: Profesionistas de ciertas clases en la entidades federativas, año de 1900," in *Estadísticas sociales del porfiriato*, 18. The urban concentration of physicians still prevailed during the 1940s. In 1940, 4.1 per cent of physicians served the rural population, which represented 58 per cent of the total population.
39 See Dr. Ismael Prieto's 1902 account of the history of the Superior Sanitation Council in José Alvarez Amézquita et al., *Historia de la salubridad,* 1: 247–52.
40 Michel Foucault, *The Birth of the Clinic: An Archaeology of Medical Perception* (London: Routledge, 1991), 31, 24–26.
41 Ibid., 34.
42 "25 Enero 1872. Ministerio de Gobernación. Reglamento del Consejo Superior de Salubridad," in Dublán and Lozano, *Legislación mexicana*, 12: 100–101.

43 "Junio 30 1879. Circular de la Secretaría de Gobernación. Organización del Consejo Superior de Salubridad," in Dublán and Lozano, *Legislación mexicana*, 13: 868–69.
44 Ibid. See also Fernando Martínez Cortés, *De los miasmas y efluvios al descubrimiento de las bacterias patógenas: Los primeros cincuenta años del Consejo Superior de Salubridad* (Mexico City: Bristol-Myers Squibb de México, 1993), 192.
45 Claudia Agostoni, "Salud pública y control social en la ciudad de México a fines del siglo diecinueve," *Historia y grafía* 17 (2001): 76–79.
46 The commissions included: schools and houses; food and beverages; theatres, temples and other places of reunion; epidemiology; dairies, slaughterhouses within the city and meat from outside the capital and all issues of sanitary police relative to animals; jails, hospitals and nursing homes; waste sites; and public works that impinged on hygiene and publications.
47 In 1880, Dr. Arellano proposed that a standard questionnaire should be made available to all the sanitary inspectors so that an efficient medical statistic could thus be formed. His proposal was approved by the President of the Republic. See *Boletín del Consejo Superior de Salubridad del Distrito Federal* 1, no. 6 (October 20 1880), 1.
48 *Boletín del Consejo Superior del Distrito Federal* 1, no. 1 (15 July 1880), 1.
49 On the hygienic education campaigns in late nineteenth century Mexico City, see Claudia Agostoni, "Discurso médico, cultura higiénica y la mujer en la ciudad de México al cambio de siglo (XIX-XX)," *Mexican Studies/Estudios Mexicanos* 18, no. 1 (Winter 2002), 1–22.
50 In Chile, President Balmaceda (1886–1891) enacted the *Ley de Policía Sanitaria* in 1886 and in 1887 the *Ordenanza General de Salubridad*, and created the Junta General de Salubridad. See Carl Murdock, "Physicians, the State and Public Health in Chile, 1881–1891," *Journal of Latin American Studies* 27 (1995): 553. In Argentina, the sanitary administration of Buenos Aires was the responsibility of the Consejo de Higiene Pública, created by the Ley 648 of the Province of Buenos Aires of 27 July 1870. In 1880, the Consejo de Higiene Pública was placed under the jurisdiction of the Departamento Nacional de Higiene, and by 1892 hygiene had become a national concern. See Salessi, *Médicos maleantes y maricas*, 33–42.
51 Alvárez Amézquita et al., *Historia de la salubridad*, 1: 327–32.
52 See "Administración Sanitaria de la Capital de la República," in *Código Sanitario de los Estados Unidos Mexicanos* (Mexico City: Imprenta del Gobierno Federal en el ex Arzobispado, 1891).
53 Alvarez Amézquita et al., *Historia de la salubridad*, 1: 330.
54 See "Libro Cuarto, artículos 349, 350 y 351" of the *Código Sanitario de los Estados Unidos Mexicanos*, reproduced in ibid, 1: 395–96.
55 Abel, *Health, Hygiene and Sanitation*, 3.
56 Alvarez Amézquita et al., *Historia de la salubridad*, 1: 402.
57 AHSS, Fondo Salubridad Pública, Epidemiología, exp. 16, caja 7.
58 Ibid.
59 Moisés González Navarro, *Población y sociedad en México (1900–1970)* (Mexico City: Universidad Nacional Autónoma de México, 1974), 1: 410.
60 *Boletín del Consejo Superior de Salubridad del Distrito Federal* 1, no. 1 (15 July 1880), 2.
61 Nancy Leys Stepan, *The Hour of Eugenics: Race, Gender and Nation in Latin America* (Ithaca, N. Y.: Cornell University Press, 1991), 25.

62 *Boletín del Consejo Superior de Salubridad del Distrito Federal* 1, no. 3 (20 September 1880), 2.
63 When the sanitary inspectors visited a home or a tenement building, they had to follow a detailed questionnaire. During the first decade of the twentieth century, the number of questions ranged between 35 and 56. The questionnaire used in 1902 can be found in AHSS, Fondo Salubridad Pública, Salubridad en el Distrito Federal, exp. 26, caja 1: "Informe de las visitas realizadas por los inspectores sanitarios a diferentes casas."
64 Until 1888, only the inoculation against smallpox was available. After 1888, a vaccine against rabies was introduced to Mexico by Eduardo Liceaga. See Ana Cecilia Rodríguez de Romo, "La ciencia pasteuriana a través de la vacuna antirrábica: el caso mexicano," *DYNAMIS* 16 (1996): 291–316.
65 "Congreso Médico. Dictamen de la Comisión de Higiene Pública," *Gaceta Médica de México* 11, no. 22 (15 November 1876), 430–36.
66 Alvarez Amézquita et al., *Historia de la salubridad*, 1: 282–85. See also "Congreso Médico," *Gaceta Médica de México* 11, no. 19 (1 October 1876): 379; and "Congreso Médico," *Gaceta Médica de México* 15, no. 20 (15 October 1876): 393–95.
67 AHCM, Policía, Salubridad, Cólera morbus, vol. 3767, exp. 34.
68 Domingo Orvañanos, "Enfermedades epidémicas y endémicas del valle de México," *Gaceta Médica de México* 29, no. 5 (March 1893): 161–63.
69 José María Reyes, "Higiene pública. Mortalidad de la niñez," *Gaceta Médica de México* 13, no. 20 (11 July 1878): 377–85.
70 AHSS, Salubridad Pública, Epidemiología, exp. 53, caja 1, and AHCM, Aguas, edificios públicos, vol. 33, exp. 152.
71 Pablo Piccato, "'El Paso de Venus,'" 217.
72 Julio Guerrero, *La génesis del crimen en México: Estudios de psiquiatría social* (Paris: Imprenta de la Viuda de Ch. Bouret, 1901).
73 González Navarro, *Historia moderna de México*, 72–82.
74 *Memoria del Consejo Superior de Salubridad*, Memoria de los trabajos ejecutados por el Consejo Superior de Salubridad en el año de 1905, Presentada por el Dr. E. Liceaga, Presidente del Consejo Superior de Salubridad al Secretario de Gobernación (Mexico City: A. Carranza y Compañía Impresores, 1905), 26.
75 José Valadés, *El Porfirismo: El crecimiento* (Mexico City: Universidad Nacional Autónoma de México, 1977), 2: 104.
76 Beezley, *Judas at the Jockey Club*, 80.
77 Prantl and Groso, *La ciudad de México*, 39.
78 Ibid., 826. On bathing, public baths and wash-houses in Mexico City during the final decades of the nineteenth century, see Agostoni, "Las delicias de la limpieza," in press.
79 Jonathan Kandell, *La Capital: The Biography of Mexico City* (New York: Random House, 1988), 388.
80 See, for instance, Hilarión Vallejo, *La penitenciaría en México desde el punto de vista de la higiene* (Mexico City: Guadalupana, 1907).
81 Diego López Rosado, *Los servicios públicos de la ciudad de México* (Mexico City: Editorial Porrúa, 1976), 219.
82 González Navarro, *Historia moderna de México*, 65–66.
83 AHCM, Policía, Salubridad, Cólera morbus, vol. 3676, exp. 31.
84 González Navarro, *Historia moderna de México*, 87–88.

85 AHCM, Consejo Superior de Gobierno del Distrito, Salubridad e higiene, vol. 646, exp. 27.
86 In 1901, the second quarter of the city had 263 streets and 1,811 houses. It was one of the most populated areas of the city and one of the poorest: Prantl and Groso, *La ciudad de México*, 691.
87 *Memoria del Consejo Superior de Salubridad, 1901*, Memoria de los trabajos ejecutados por el Consejo Superior de Salubridad en el año de 1901 (Mexico City: Imprenta de Eduardo Dublán, 1902), 44.
88 Ibid., 77.
89 Ibid., 76.
90 AHCM, Policía, Salubridad, Epidemias, vol. 3675, exp. 24.
91 Ibid., and AHCM, Consejo Superior de Gobierno del Distrito, Salubridad e higiene, vol. 645, exp. 16.
92 *Memoria del Consejo Superior de Salubridad,* 1905, 65.
93 Alan Knight, "Revolutionary Project, Recalcitrant People: Mexico, 1910–1940," in *The Revolutionary Process in Mexico: Essays on Political and Social Change, 1880–1940*, edited by Jaime E. Rodríguez (Los Angeles: UCLA, Latin American Center Publications, 1990), 238.
94 *Memoria del Consejo Superior de Salubridad*, 1905, 66.
95 Ibid., 68.
96 AHCM, Consejo Superior de Gobierno del Distrito, Salubridad e higiene, vol. 646, exp. 27.
97 *Memoria del Consejo Superior de Salubridad*, 1905, 68.
98 Ibid., 99.
99 Ibid.
100 Ibid., 102.
101 See Juan Breña, "Sobre algunas prácticas religiosas que deben abolirse en beneficio de la higiene," in *Memoria General del IV Congreso Médico Nacional Mexicano efectuado en la ciudad de México del 9 al 25 de septiembre de 1910* (año del Centenario), (Mexico City: Tipografía Económica, 1910), 674–81; and José Guillermo Salazar, "Supersticiones y creencias vulgares en los países de Hispano-América," in *Memoria de la Sociedad Científica 'Antonio Alzate': Revista Científica y Bibliográfica* 32, nos. 5–9 (1911–1912): 427–33.
102 Hira de Gortari, "¿Un modelo de urbanización? La ciudad de México a finales del siglo XIX," *Secuencia* 8, Revista Americana de Ciencias Sociales (January–April 1987): 45.
103 AHCM, Policía, Salubridad, Cólera morbus, vol. 3676, exp. 37.

Notes to Chapter 4

1 "El arte y la historia: manía de estatuas," *El Universal*, 6 August 1892.
2 Gareth A. Jones and Anne Varley, "The Contest of the City Centre: Street Traders versus Buildings," *Bulletin of Latin American Research* 13, no. 1 (1994): 27–44. See also Edward Soja and B. Hooper, "The Spaces that Difference Makes: Some Notes on the Geographical Margins of the New Cultural Policies," in *Place and Politics of Identity*, edited by Michael Keith and Steve Pile (London: Routledge, 1993), 183–84.
3 Jan Bazant, "From Independence to the Liberal Republic, 1821–1867," in *Mexico Since Independence*, edited by Leslie Bethell (Cambridge: Cambridge University Press, 1991), 39–40.

4 Israel Katzman, *Arquitectura del siglo XIX en México* (Mexico City: Trillas, 1988), 18.
5 According to the historian Luis González Obregón, the first monument to Independence was provisional and consisted of a sculpture of the national emblem, placed upon the statue of Charles IV on 27 October 1821, when this statue stood in the center of the Plaza Mayor. See "La Jura de la Independencia," *El Mundo Ilustrado*, 16 September 1905. The first monument to Independence was made in Celaya, Guanajuato, in 1822. In 1843, Lorenzo de la Hidalga's project for a monument to Independence was planned for the Plaza Mayor. The monument was begun that same year, but the only piece of the monument erected on the Plaza Mayor was the base or *"zócalo,"* and since then the Plaza Mayor or Plaza de la Constitución has been commonly referred to as *"Zócalo."*
6 *El Siglo XIX*, 13 August 1862.
7 The Castle of Chapultepec was build by orders of Viceroy Bernardo de Gálves in 1785. Regarding the remodelling of the castle during Maximilian's Empire, see Michael Drewes, "Proyecto de remodelación del Palacio de Chapultepec en la época del Emperador Maximiliano," *Anales del Instituto de Investigaciones Estéticas* 51 (1983): 73–82.
8 See the newspaper *La Sociedad,* 17 September 1865. Quoted in Alfonso Alcocer, *La columna de la Independencia* (Mexico City: Ediciones de la Delegación Cuauhtémoc, Departamento del Distrito Federal, n.d.), 10.
9 The monument to Charles IV was designed in 1802 by the Spaniard Manuel Tolsá. For a detailed analysis of the role of Francisco Somera's involvement in the expansion of the city, see María Dolores Morales, "Francisco Somera y el primer fraccionamiento de la ciudad de México," in *Formación y desarrollo de la burguesía en México*, edited by Ciro Cardoso (Mexico: Siglo XXI, 1978), 188–230.
10 For an analysis of the urban transformation of Paris during Eugène Haussmann's 17 years as Prefect of the city, see David Pinkney, *Napoleon III and the Rebuilding of Paris* (Princeton, NJ: Princeton University Press, 1958), and Pierre Lavedán, *Histoire de l'urbanisme: Epoque contemporaine*, vol. 3 (Paris: Henri Laurens, 1952).
11 According to Barbara Tenenbaum, the source of inspiration for the new paseo was Vienna, not Paris. See Barbara Tenenbaum, "Murals in Stone: The Paseo de la Reforma and Porfirian Mexico, 1873–1910," in *La ciudad y el campo en la historia de México. Papers presented at the VII Conference of Mexican and the United States Historians, Oaxaca, 1985* (Mexico City: Universidad Nacional Autónoma de México, 1992), 1: 369. Also see Mauricio Gómez Mayorga, "La influencia francesa en la arquitectura y el urbanismo en México," in *La intervención francesa y el Imperio de Maximiliano cien años después, 1862–1962*, edited by Arturo Arnáiz y Freg and Claude Bataillon (Mexico City: Asociación Mexicana de Historiadores – Instituto Francés de América Latina, 1965), 185. Also see Carl E. Schorske, *Fin-de-siècle Vienna: Politics and Culture* (New York: Vintage Books, 1981).
12 Francis Violich, "Mexico City and Mexico: Two Cultural Worlds in Perspective," *Third World Planning Review* 3, no. 4 (1983): 369–79. Also see AHCM, Paseo de la Reforma, vol. 3585, exp. 2.
13 Tenenbaum, "Murals in Stone," 370.

14 For instance, see Hubert Howe Bancroft, *Resources and Development of Mexico* (San Francisco: The Bancroft Company Publishers, 1893); Henry C. Becher, *A Trip to Mexico* (Toronto: Willing and Williamson, 1880); Fanny Chambers Gooch, *Face to Face with the Mexicans* (New York: Howard and Hulbert, 1887); Gustave Gostkowsky, *De Paris à Mexico par les Etat Unis* (Paris: P. V. Stock Editeur, 1889); and Adolfo Dollero, *México al día, impresiones y notas de viaje* (Mexico City: Librería Vda. de C. Bouret, 1911).
15 Some guides to the city included: *Almanaque Bouret para el año de 1897*, Formado bajo la dirección de Raúl Mille y Alberto Leduc (Mexico City: Instituto de Investigaciones Dr. José María Luis Mora, 1992); Reau Campbells, *Campbell's New Revised Complete Guide and Descriptive Book of Mexico* (Chicago: Roger and Smith Co., 1909); J. Figueroa Domenech, *Guía general descriptiva de la República Mexicana* (Mexico City: Araluce, 1889); Emil Riedel, *Practical Guide of the City and Valley of Mexico* (Mexico City: J. Epstein, 1892); and Manuel Tornel, *Guía práctica del viajero y del comerciante en México* (Mexico City: Librería de la Enseñanza, 1876).
16 See Rita Eder, "La fotografía en México en el siglo XIX," *Historia del arte mexicano*, vol. 9 (Mexico City: Secretaría de Educación Pública – Instituto Nacional de Bellas Artes – Salvat, 1982); Francisco Montellano, *C.B. Waite, fotógrafo: Una mirada diversa sobre el México de principios de siglo* (Mexico City: Grijalbo, 1994); and Rosa Casanova and Olivier Debroise, *Sobre la superficie bruñida de un espejo* (Mexico City: Fondo de Cultura Económica, 1989).
17 Robert Levine, "Images of Progress in Nineteenth-Century Latin America," *Journal of Urban History* 15, no. 3 (May 1989): 310.
18 Prantl and Groso, *La ciudad de México*, 690.
19 Clementina Díaz y de Ovando, "La ciudad de México en 1904," *Historia Mexicana* 24 (1974): 123.
20 Berta Tello Peón, "Intención decorativa en los objetos de uso cotidiano de los interiores domésticos del porfiriato," in *El arte y la vida cotidiana: XVI Coloquio Internacional de Historia del Arte* (Mexico City: Instituto de Investigaciones Estéticas, UNAM, 1995), 139–54.
21 Katzman, *Arquitectura del siglo XIX*, 138. See also *The Concise Oxford Dictionary of Art and Artists*, edited by I. Chilvers (Oxford: Oxford University Press, 1992), 144.
22 For a thorough analysis of the stylistic diversity in Mexico City's architecture during the Porfiriato, see Katzman, *Arquitectura del siglo XIX*, 138–39, 157–59, 199–209, 229, 239–48, 256, 266–67. Also see the following studies of public and residential architecture in Mexico City: Antonio Boret Correa, "La arquitectura de la época Porfiriana en México," *Anales de la Universidad de Murcia* 24 (1965–1966): 249–309; Vicente Martín Hernández, *Arquitectura doméstica de la Ciudad de México, 1890–1925* (Mexico City: Escuela de Arquitectura – UNAM, 1981); and Juan Urquiaga, *Arquitectura en México: porfiriato y movimiento moderno* (Mexico City: INBA, 1983).
23 Steven Topik, "Economic Domination by the Capital: Mexico City and Rio de Janeiro, 1888–1910," in *La ciudad y el campo en la historia de México: Papers presented at the VII Conference of Mexican and the United States Historians*, Oaxaca, 1985 (Mexico City: Universidad Nacional Autónoma de México, 1992), 1: 192.
24 Ibid.

25 Gustavo Garza, "El sistema ferroviario y eléctrico como génesis de la concentración industrial en la ciudad de México (1876–1910)," in *La ciudad y el campo en la historia de México: Papers presented at the VII Conference of Mexican and the United States Historians, Oaxaca, 1985* (Mexico City: Universidad Nacional Autónoma de México, 1992), 1: 242.
26 Diego López Rosado, *Historia y pensamiento económico en México: Finanzas públicas – obras públicas* (Mexico City: Universidad Nacional Autónoma de México, 1972), 148.
27 For instance, see Garza, "El sistema ferroviario," 215–46; Victor Manuel Durand Ponte, *México: La formación de un país dependiente* (Mexico City: Instituto de Investigaciones Sociales – Universidad Nacional Autónoma de México, 1979); David M. Pletcher, *Rails, Mines and Progress* (Port Washington: Kennikat, 1972); and Luis Unikel, *La dinámica del crecimiento de la ciudad de México* (Mexico City: Fundación para Estudios de la Población, A.C., 1972).
28 Dawn Ades, *Art in Latin America: The Modern Era, 1820–1980* (London: The Hayward Gallery, 1986), 106.
29 Carlos Monsiváis, "La aparición del subsuelo. Sobre la cultura de la Revolución Mexicana," *Historias 8–9: Nuevas Reflexiones sobre la Revolución Mexicana* (Mexico City: Instituto Nacional de Antropología e Historia, 1985), 171.
30 Antonio Peñafiel, *Explicación del edificio mexicano para la Exposición Internacional de París en 1889* (Mexico City: 1889), 53. See the thorough analysis of the World's Fairs from 1851 to 1939 made by Paul Greenhalgh, *Ephemeral Vistas: The Expositions Universelles, Great Exhibitions and World's Fairs, 1851–1939* (Manchester: Manchester University Press, 1988). With regard to Mexico's participation in World's Fairs, see Mauricio Tenorio Trillo, *Mexico at World's Fairs: Crafting a Modern Nation* (California: Berkeley, 1997).
31 Sonia Lombardo de Ruiz, *El pasado prehispánico en la cultura nacional (Memoria hemerográfica, 1877–1911): El Monitor Republicano (1877–1896)* (Mexico City: Instituto Nacional de Antropología e Historia – Antologías Serie Historia, 1994), 1: 24.
32 A recent display of Mexican art as propaganda for the political stability and economic progress of the country took place in 1990 in the Metropolitan Museum of Art, New York, with the largest exhibition of Mexican art ever shown in the United States, the exhibition "Mexico: Splendors of Thirty Centuries." On this exhibition, see Roger Bartra, "Mexican Oficio: The Miseries and Splendors of Culture," *Third Text* 14 (1991): 7–16.
33 The United States became the most significant catalyst for debate on the question of identity during the Porfiriato, a debate that took place in the midst of a climate of rapid economic development. Justo Sierra sought to find the "Mexican" social origins in the "mestizo" family. See Hale, *Transformation of Liberalism*, 253–54, and Justo Sierra, *Evolución política del pueblo Mexicano*, Obras Completas del Maestro Justo Sierra (Mexico City: Universidad Nacional Autónoma de México, 1957), 13: 56, 98.
34 Horst Woldemar Janson, *Nineteenth-Century Sculpture* (London: Thames and Hudson, 1985),176. Also see Eric Hobsbawm, "Mass Producing Traditions: Europe, 1870–1914," in *The Invention of Tradition*, edited by Eric Hobsbawm and Terrence Ranger (London: Canto, 1995), 263–307.

35 Helen Escobedo's Foreword to *Mexican Monuments, Strange Encounters* (New York: Abbeville Press, 1989), 8.

36 Ibid. See also *Les lieux de mémoire 1: La République*, edited by Pierre Nora (Paris: Bibliothèque illustrée des histories – Gallimard, 1984), for a thorough analysis of the monumental endeavour in France. For Brazil, see José Murilho de Carvalho, *A forma ão das almas: O imaginario da República no Brasil* (São Paulo: Companhia das Letras 1990). For Buenos Aires, see María Teresa Espantoso Rodríguez et al., "Imágenes para la Nación Argentina: Conformación de un eje monumental urbano en Buenos Aires entre 1811 y 1910," in *Arte, Historia e Identidad en América: Visiones Comparativas. XVII Coloquio Internacional de Historia del Arte* (Mexico City: Instituto de Investigaciones Estéticas, Universidad Nacional Autónoma de México, 1994), 345–60.

37 Tenenbaum, "Murals in Stone," 370, 372.

38 Ibid., 371.

39 Justino Fernández, *El arte del siglo XIX en México* (Mexico City: Imprenta Universitaria, 1967), 167, my italics. See also Francisco Sosa, *Apuntamiento para la historia del Monumento a Cuauhtémoc* (Mexico City: Oficina Tipográfica de la Secretaría de Fomento, 1887).

40 Fernández, *El arte del siglo XIX*, 171. The statue of Columbus is supported by a pedestal that has two bas-reliefs, one depicting his arrival in America, the other the construction of a church. In the corners of the pedestal, the statues of fray--?friar?-- Juan de Torquemada, fray Pedro de Gante, fray Bartolomé de Olmedo and fray Bartolomé de las Casas surround Columbus.

41 Ibid., 170–73; Tenenbaum, "Murals in Stone," 370; and Barbara Tenenbaum, "Streetwise History: The Paseo de la Reforma and the Porfirian State, 1876–1910," in *Rituals of Rule, Rituals of Resistance: Public Celebrations and Popular Culture in Mexico*, edited by William Beezley, Cheryl English Martin and William E. French (Wilmington: Scholarly Resources, 1994), 131.

42 Eric Hobsbawm, *The Age of Empire, 1875–1914* (London: Abacus, 1995), 27.

43 Clementina Díaz y de Ovando's Foreword to *Vicente Riva Palacio: Cuentos del General* (Mexico City: Editorial Porrúa, 1986), xix-xxi.

44 Francisco Sosa, *Las estatuas de la Reforma: notas biográficas de los personajes en ellas representados* (Mexico City: Oficina Tipográfica de la Secretaría de Fomento, 1900), 33–34. The first edition of this text was published in French and sent to the Paris *Exposition Universelle* of 1900. In it, a full list of the statues and biographical information of all the heroes can be found. Also see Joe Nash, *El Paseo de la Reforma: A Guide* (Mexico City: Raul Esquivel, 1959), 27–87.

45 Manuel Gutiérrez Nájera, *Escritos inéditos de sabor satírico "Platos del día,"* (Columbia, Missouri: University of Missouri Press, 1972), 37.

46 Tenenbaum, "Murals in Stone," 378. Also see Sosa, *Apuntamiento para la historia;* and Angélica Velázquez-Guadarrama, "La historia patria en el Paseo de la Reforma: La propuesta de Francisco Sosa y la consolidación del estado en el Porfiriato," in *Estudios de Arte y Estética 37. XVII Coloquio Internacional de Historia del Arte. Arte, Historia e Identidad en América: Visiones Comparativas* (Mexico City: Instituto de Investigaciones Estéticas – Universidad Nacional Autónoma de México, 1994), 333–44. Also see AHCM, Gobierno del Distrito, Obras públicas, vol. 1761, exp. 968, for a report that details the inauguration of the statues in the Paseo de la Reforma of General Ignácio

Rayón and Francisco Manuel Sánchez de Tagle donated by the state of Michoacán in 1899.

47 See *El Universal*, 6 August 1892. Among other statues placed in the city were two bronze statues representing Jupiter and Venus in the Alameda, and one of Doña Josefa Ortíz de Domínguez — *La Corregidora* (1768–1829) — erected on the Plaza de Santo Domingo in Mexico City and unveiled in 1900. In other states of the Republic monuments were also erected, such as the statue of General Ignacio Zaragoza in Puebla; of General Ramón Corona in Guadalajara and one of Benito Juárez in Chihuahua.

48 Daniel Schávelzon, "El primer monumento a Cuauhtémoc (1869)," in *La polémica del arte nacional en México, 1850–1910*, edited by Daniel Schávelzon (Mexico City: Fondo de Cultura Económica, 1988), 109–11. For detailed information regarding this monument, see "Proyecto para erigir una estatua al Emperador Azteca Cuauhtémoc en la glorieta de Jamaica en el Paseo de la Viga," and "Programa de la Inauguración del Monumento a Guautimotzin en el Paseo de la Viga," AHCM, Historia, Monumentos, vol. 2276, exp. 17. Also see Antonio García Cubas, *Geografía e historia del Distrito Federal*, Facsimile of the 1894 edition (Mexico City: Instituto de Investigaciones Dr. José María Luis Mora, 1993), 81.

49 Fernández, *El arte del siglo XIX*, 168. Engineer Jiménez also made a monument to Hidalgo in the state of Chihuahua and a relief monument in honour of Enrico Martínez — the author of the project of the drainage of the valley of Mexico in the seventeenth century — which was to stand opposite the Palacio Nacional. The project for the 'Monumento Hidrográfico' to honour Enrico Martínez's struggle against the flooding of the city was approved by President Díaz on 23 July 1877. See "Bases para la erección del Monumento Hidrográfico," AHCM, Historia, Monumentos, vol. 2276, exp. 26. See also Antonio García Cubas, *Atlas geográfico y estadístico de los Estados Unidos Mexicanos* (Mexico City: Oficina Tipográfica de la Secretaría de Fomento, 1884), 80.

50 *Memoria de Fomento* 1877–1882, 3: 332–33, quoted in Tenenbaum, "Murals in Stone," 374.

51 "Notas sobre Manuel Vilar y sus esculturas de Moctezuma y Tlahuicole," in *La polémica del arte nacional en México, 1850–1910*, edited by Daniel Schávelzon (Mexico City: Fondo de Cultura Económica, 1988), 81.

52 Ida Rodríguez Prampolini, "La figura del indio en la pintura del siglo XIX: fondo ideológico," in *La polémica del arte nacional en México, 1850–1910*, edited by Daniel Schávelzon (Mexico City: Fondo de Cultura Económica, 1988), 205.

53 Ibid., 211.

54 Ibid., 204. Leandro Izaguirre's *Torture of Cuauhtémoc* (1893) was a gigantic canvas made for the Chicago World Fair held in 1893. It symbolized national resistance and portrayed the heroic figure of Cuauhtémoc confronting the Spanish invader.

55 Sosa, *Apuntamiento para la historia*, 3, 20; and Vicente Reyes in the *Anales de la Asociación de Ingenieros y Arquitectos* 1, 1887,Reproduced in "Notas sobre Manuel Vilar y sus esculturas de Moctezuma y Tlahuicole," in *La polémica del arte nacional*, 115.

56 The full program of activities set out for the inauguration of Cuauhtémoc's monument can be found in Josefina García Quintana, *Cuauhtémoc en el siglo*

XIX (Mexico City: Instituto de Investigaciones Históricas – Universidad Nacional Autónoma de México, 1977). See her appendix: *Diario del Hogar: Periódico de las Familias*, 21 August 1887.
57 Marina Warner, *Monuments and Maidens: The Allegory of the Female Form* (London: Picador, 1985), 127–28.
58 Carlos Monsiváis, "On Civic Monuments and their Spectators," in *Mexican Monuments; Strange Encounters*, edited by Helen Escobedo (New York: Abbeville Press, 1989), 118.
59 Itzcóatl was the fourth Aztec king (1428–1440), and Ahuítzotl was the eighth Aztec king (1486–1503) and father of Cuauhtémoc.
60 *El Universal*, 6 August 1892.
61 Prantl and Groso, *La ciudad de México*, 703.
62 *El Imparcial*, 4 March 1900.
63 AHCM, Consejo Superior de Gobierno del Distrito, Salubridad e higiene, vol. 645, exp. 13.
64 Prantl and Groso, *La ciudad de México*, 450.
65 AHCM, Aguas, arquerías y acueductos, vol. 18, exp. 169.
66 Ibid., vol. 18, exp. 187 and exp. 195.
67 Ibid., vol. 18, exp. 204.
68 Ibid. For a detailed history of the aqueducts in Mexico City, see Alain Musset, *De l'eau vive à l'eau morte: Enjeux techniques et culturels dans la vallée de Mexico (XVIe-XIXe siècles)* (Paris: Editions Recherche sur les Civilisations, 1991), 111–39.
69 AHCM, Consejo Superior de Gobierno del Distrito, Salubridad e higiene, vol. 645, exp. 9.
70 Ibid., exp. 12.
71 "Proyecto de reglamento de las fábricas, industrias, depósitos y demas establecimientos peligrosos, insalubres é incomodos," *Boletín del Consejo Superior de Salubridad del Distrito Federal* 3, nos. 1–2 (31 August 1882). Also see Alvarez Amézquita et al., *Historia de la salubridad*, 1: 360–73.
72 Charles Weeks, *The Juárez Myth in Mexico* (Alabama: University of Alabama Press, 1987), 27.
73 An "invented traditions" is taken to mean "a set of practices, normally governed by overtly or tacitly accepted rules and of a ritual or symbolic nature, which seek to inculcate certain values and norms of behavior by repetition, which automatically implies a continuity with the past ... where possible, they normally attempt to establish continuity with a suitable historic past ... insofar as there is such reference to a historic past, the peculiarity of 'invented' traditions is that the continuity within it is largely factitious." See Hobsbawm and Ranger, *The Invention of Tradition* (London: Canto, 1995), 1–2.
74 Weeks, *Juárez Myth in Mexico*, 28.
75 Mauricio Tenorio Trillo, "1910 Mexico City: Space and Nation in the City of the Centenario," *Journal of Latin American Studies* 28, pt. 1 (February 1996): 96–97.
76 Weeks, *Juárez Myth in México*, 1.
77 "Informe leído por el señor Diputado é Ingeniero don Ignacio L. de la Barra en el acto de la inauguración del monumento á Benito Juárez, el 18 de septiembre de 1910," reproduced in Genaro García, *Crónica oficial de las*

fiestas del primer Centenario de la Independencia de México, 1911(Mexico City: Facsimile edition, Centro de Estudios de Historia de México, 1991), 79.
78 Ibid.
79 "Discurso pronunciado por el señor Licenciado don Carlos Robles en el acto de la inauguración del monumento á Benito Juárez, el 18 de septiembre de 1910," reproduced in ibid., 81.
80 Hale, *Transformation of Liberalism*, 24.
81 Tenorio Trillo,"1910 Mexico City," 96–97.
82 "Discurso pronunciado por el señor Licenciado don Carlos Robles ...," reproduced in García, *Crónica oficial de las fiestas*, 80; and "Informe leído por el señor Diputado e Ingeniero don Ignacio L. de la Barra," reproduced in ibid., 79.
83 Tenorio Trillo, "1910 Mexico City," 95. Also see Tenenbaum, "Streetwise History," 146.
84 The winged victory became the visible manifestation of triumph. For instance, in New York ,sculptor Saint-Gaudens' Victory leading General Sherman by the rein was completed in 1900 and erected in 1903. Ettore Ximenes crowned the Palazzo di Giustizia in Rome with a winged victory at the turn of the century. In 1911, the gilded Victory on the pinnacle of the Victoria Monument in the Mall in London by Thomas Brock was unveiled. See Warner, *Monuments and Maidens*, 143.
85 See Jesús Galindo y Villa, "Lugar en que debe colocarse el monumento á la Independencia Nacional," reproduced in Alcocer, *La columna de la independencia*, 65–66.
86 *El Imparcial*, 16 September 1910.
87 Alcocer, *La columna de la independencia*, 39.
88 See the description of the monument written by its architect, Antonio Rivas Mercado: "Informe leído por el señor Ingeniero don Antonio Rivas Mercado, Director de la Escuela Nacional de Bellas Artes, en el acto de la inauguración de la Columna de la Independencia, el 16 de septiembre de 1910," reproduced in García, *Crónica oficial de las fiestas*, 74–75.
89 Fernández, *El arte del siglo XIX*, 175.
90 Warner, *Monuments and Maidens*, 128–31.
91 "Discurso pronunciado por el señor Licenciado don Miguel S. Macedo. Subsecretario de Gobernación, en el acto de la inauguración de la Columna de la Independencia, el 16 de septiembre de 1910," reproduced en García, *Crónica oficial de las fiestas*, 77.
92 Sierra, *Evolución política del pueblo*, 361–69.
93 Rita Eder, "The Icons of Power and Popular Art," in *Mexican Monuments, Strange Encounters*, edited by Helen Escobedo (New York: Abbeville Press, 1989), 65–66. Also see Ilene Virginia O'Malley, *The Myth of the Revolution: Hero Cults and the Institutionalization of the Mexican State, 1920–1940* (New York: Greenwood Press, 1986).
94 "'Al Buen Cura,' Poesía recitada por el señor Diputado don Salvador Díaz Mirón en el acto de la inauguración de la Columna de la Independencia, el 16 de septiembre de 1910," reproduced en García, *Crónica oficial de las fiestas,* 78.
95 "Discurso pronunciado por el señor Licenciado don Miguel S. Macedo, Subsecretario de Gobernación, en el acto de la inauguración de la Columna de la Independencia, el 16 de septiembre de 1910," reproduced in ibid., 77.

96 For a detailed account of the activities of the Comisión Nacional del Centenario and of all the events, inaugurations, parades and other activities that took place in Mexico City, see García, *Crónica oficial de las fiestas*. See also Tenorio Trillo, *Mexico at the World's Fairs*.
97 AHSS, Salubridad en el Distrito Federal, exp. 1, caja 2: *Informes de los kioskos sanitarios en mal estado en los cuarteles de la Ciudad de México*.
98 Ibid.
99 Ibid.
100 Ibid.
101 AHCM, Consejo Superior de Gobierno del Distrito, Salubridad e higiene, vol. 646, exp. 23.
102 Ibid.
103 Ibid., exp. 26.
104 Ibid.
105 This proposal was made by E. Lozano, R. Nervo, Carlos Lazo de la Vega and R. Riveroll del Prado.
106 García, "Exposición Popular de Higiene," in *Crónica oficial de las fiestas*, 262.
107 Charles Flandrau, *Viva Mexico! A Traveller's Account of Life in Mexico* (London: Eland, 1990), 282.

Notes to Chapter 5

1 See Goubert, *Conquest of Water*, 25.
2 Stanley K. Schultz and Clay McShane, "To Engineer the Metropolis: Sewers, Sanitation, and City Planning in Late-Nineteenth-Century America," *Journal of American History* 65, no. 2 (September 1978): 389.
3 A. Mille, *Assainissement des villes par l'eau, les égouts, les irrigations* (Paris: 1885), quoted in Donald Reid, *Paris Sewers and Sewermen: Realities and Representations* (Cambridge Massachusetts: Harvard University Press, 1991), 35–36, 58.
4 Mílada Bazant, "La enseñanza y la práctica de la ingeniería durante el Porfiriato," *Historia Mexicana* 3 (1984): 254–297.
5 Musset, *De l'eau vive à l'eau morte*, 225–73, where he stresses the importance of water for the Aztecs, what he calls "les civilisations de l'eau."
6 The project belonged to Francisco Gudiel and Ruy González and emerged after the flood of October 1555, which reduced the traffic of the city to canoes and caused the collapse of numerous houses. The proposal, made on 26 November, argued that the only way the city of New Spain could be saved was by draining the water of the lakes and expelling it from the valley of Mexico. See *Memoria de las obras del sistema del drenaje profundo del Distrito Federal* (Mexico City: Departamento del Distrito Federal, 1975) 2: 86–90; and Musset, *De l'eau vive à l'eau morte*, 313–18.
7 Louisa Hoberman, "Bureaucracy and Disaster: Mexico City and the Flood of 1629," *Journal of Latin American Studies* 6 (1974): 212. For a detailed analysis of the 1607 project and subsequent projects up to 1855, see Luis González Obregón, "Reseña histórica del desagüe del Valle de México 1449–1855," in *Memoria histórica, técnica y administrativa de las Obras del Desagüe del Valle de México, 1449–1900, publicada por orden de la Junta Directiva del mismo Desagüe* (Mexico City: Tipografía de la Oficina Impresora de Estampillas, Palacio Nacional, 1902).

8. Hoberman, "Bureaucracy and Disaster," 212–13.
9. The prolific life of Enrico Martínez has been studied by Francisco de la Maza. See his book *Enrico Martínez, cosmógrafo e impresor de la Nueva España* (Mexico City: Sociedad Mexicana de Geografía y Estadística, 1943).
10. Hoberman, "Bureaucracy and Disaster," 212–13.
11. Michael W. Mathes, "To save a city: the desagüe of Mexico-Huehuetoca, 1607," *The Americas* 26 (1970): 437. For an account of the destruction experienced in the city following the 1629 flood, see Francisco de la Maza, Maza, *La ciudad de México en el siglo XVII* (Mexico City: Fondo de Cultura Económica, 1968), 26–28.
12. Hoberman, "Bureaucracy and Disaster," 214. Also see Roberto Ríos Elizondo, *Apuntes para una historia de las inundaciones de la ciudad de México* (Mexico City: Boletín de la Sociedad Mexicana de Geografía y Estadística, 1954), 319.
13. The proposal to abandon the city was first formulated in 1555 after a flood destroyed much of the city. However, as in 1630, it was rejected by the Viceroy and by the inhabitants of the city, who argued that much had already been invested in the capital of New Spain.
14. Hoberman, "Bureaucracy and Disaster," 225; González Obregón, "Reseña histórica del desagüe del Valle de México 1449–1855," 1: 235–47; and Musset, *De l'eau vive à l'eau morte*, 66–67. The *Códice Florentino*, book 1, plate VII, illustrates the place where the mythical *sumidero* was located: "Representación del lugar en medio de la laguna, llamado Pantitlán, donde se encontraba el sumidero."
15. Hoberman, "Bureaucracy and Disaster," 222.
16. Ibid., 228.
17. An important study of the drainage system of Huehuetoca was made by Jorge Gurría Lacroix, *El desagüe del valle de México durante la época novohispana* (Mexico City: Universidad Nacional Autónoma de México, 1978). See also Charles Gibson, *The Aztecs Under Spanish Rule: A History of the Indians of the Valley of Mexico, 1519–1810* (Stanford California: Stanford University Press, 1964), 236–56, where he analyzes the colonial efforts to protect the city and how labour was organized for the drainage works.
18. González Obregón, "Reseña histórica del desagüe," 1: 526.
19. See José María Luis Mora, *Memoria que para informar sobre el origen y estado actual de las obras emprendidas para el desagüe de las lagunas del valle de México, presentó a la Excma. Diputación Provincial el Vocal Dr. D. José María Luis Mora, comisionado para reconocerlas* (Mexico City: Imprenta de la Aguila, 1823); and Ernesto Lemoine Villicaña, *El desagüe del Valle de México durante la época Independiente* (Mexico City: Instituto de Investigaciones Históricas – Universidad Nacional Autónoma de México, 1978), 51–52.
20. Alejandro de Humboldt, *Ensayo político sobre el reino de la Nueva España*, Estudio preliminar, revisión del texto, notas y anexos de Juan Antonio Ortega y Medina (Mexico City: Editorial Porrúa, 1966), 149–50.
21. González Obregón, "Reseña histórica del desagüe," 1: 228.
22. Lemoine Villicaña, *El desagüe del Valle de México*, 52.
23. Luis Espinosa, "Reseña histórica y técnica de las obras del desagüe del valle de México, 1856–1900," in *Memoria histórica, técnica y administrativa de las Obras del Desagüe del Valle de México. 1449–1900*, publicada por orden de la Junta Directiva del mismo Desagüe (Mexico City: Tipografía de la Oficina Impresora de Estampillas, Palacio Nacional, 1902), 1: 281–82.

24 Claudia Agostoni, "Mexican Hygienists and the Political and Economic Elite during the Porfirio Díaz regime. The Case of Mexico City (1876–1910)," in *Les Hygiénistes, Enjeux, modèles et pratiques (XVIIIe–XXe siècles)*, sous la direction de Patrice Bourdelais (Paris: Éditions Belin, 2001), 193–210.

25 *Brief Sketch of the Drainage Works of the Valley of Mexico*, Written expressly for the delegates of the Pan-American Congress (Mexico City: Tipografía de Francisco Díaz de León, 1901).

26 *Memoria histórica, técnica y administrativa de las obras del desagüe del valle de México, 1449–1900*. Publicada por orden de la Junta Directiva del mismo Desagüe, 3 vols (Mexico: Tipografía de la Oficina Impresora de Estampillas, Palacio Nacional, 1902).

27 See Espinosa, "Reseña histórica y técnica ," 1: 359–60.

28 González Navarro, *Historia moderna de México*, 123.

29 "Ingeniería Sanitaria. Comisión de atargeas del Consejo Superior de Salubridad, 20 May 1881,"quoted in Alvarez Amézquita et al., *Historia de la salubridad*, 1: 306–7.

30 Ibid., 1: 308–9 and 317.

31 AHCM. Desagüe, vol. 745, exp. 113.

32 Ibid.

33 Ibid.

34 AHCM, Policía. Salubridad, Cólera morbus, vol. 3676, exp. 34.

35 *La salubridad é higiene pública en los Estados Unidos Mexicanos. Brevísima reseña de los progresos alcanzados desde 1810 hasta 1910. Publicada por el Consejo Superior de Salubridad, bajo cuyos auspicios tuvo á bien poner la Secretaría de Estado y del Despacho de Gobernación las Conferencias y la Exposición Popular de Higiene, con las cuales se sirvió contribuir a la celebración del Primer Centenario de la Independencia Nacional. Año del Centenario, 1910* (Mexico City: Casa Metodista de Publicaciones, 1910), lxxxix. See also Manuel Perló Cohen, *El paradigma porfiriano. Historia del desagüe del valle de México* (Mexico City: Porrúa, 1999).

36 Lemoine Villicaña, *El desagüe del Valle de México*, 93–94.

37 See Rosendo Esparza, "Reseña administrativa y económica de la Junta Directiva del Desagüe del valle de México, 1886–1900," in *Memoria histórica, técnica y administrativa de las Obras del Desagüe del Valle de México, 1449–1900, publicada por orden de la Junta Directiva del mismo Desagüe* (Mexico City: Tipografía de la Oficina Impresora de Estampillas, Palacio Nacional, 1902), 1: 530.

38 *El Tiempo*, 16 July 1886.

39 Moíses González Navarro, "México en una laguna," *Historia Mexicana* 4 (1955): 506–10.

40 AHCM. Historia. Inundaciones, vol. 2275, exp. 2.

41 Ibid., exp. 10.

42 Ibid., exp. 12.

43 *Memoria histórica, técnica y administrativa de las Obras del Desagüe del Valle de México, 1449–1900*, 1: ix.

44 Luis Espinosa and Isidro Díaz Lombardo, "Reseña técnica de la ejecución del Gran Canal, y de las obras de arte, 1886–1900," in *Memoria histórica, técnica y administrativa de las Obras del Desagüe del Valle de México, 1449–1900, publicada por orden de la Junta Directiva del mismo Desagüe* (Mexico City: Tipografía de la Oficina Impresora de Estampillas, Palacio Nacional, 1902), 1: 518.

45 Esparza, "Reseña administrativa y económica," 1: 556. In particular, see Priscilla Connolly, *El contratista de Don Porfirio. Obras públicas, deuda y desarrollo desigual* (Mexico City: Fondo de Cultura Económica, 1997).
46 Esparza, "Reseña administrativa y económica," 1: 556–57. Also see Jonathan Brown, "Foreign and Native-Born Workers in Porfirian México," *The American Historical Review* 98, no. 3 (1993): 786–818, who compares the conditions of Mexican and foreign workers in the rail and mining industries in northern Mexico during the Porfiriato.
47 The original contract between the Junta Directiva del Desagüe del Valle de México and Pearson & Sons can be found in Science Museum Archive, London (SMA), Records of S. Pearson & Sons (PEA) Box 16/1. The British firm Pearson and Sons was founded in Bradford Yorkshire in 1856, and established its reputation in the 1880s with a succession of major engineering works throughout the world, such as the Sheffield Main Sewer, the docks at Halifax, Canada, the Blackwall Tunnel and Dover Harbour, as well as the Sennar Dam on the Blue Nile. In Mexico, it responsible not only for the Gran Canal of the drainage works for the valley and city of Mexico, but also the reconstruction of the Tehuantepec Railway and Port 1902–1907, as well as Veracruz Harbour, 1895–1902, among others. See also Connolly, *El contratista de Don Porfirio*, 17–44, 280–304.
48 The description by John Body of the functioning of the drainage works and in particular that of the Gran Canal is as follows: "The present works consist of a Canal, commencing at the San Lázaro Gate of the City, and has a total length of 47,580 meters. For the first 20 kilometers it runs between the Guadalupe Hills and Lake Texcoco in a northeast direction, with a width at the bottom of five meters, and an average depth of 9 meters. This section is only intended to take water and sewerage of the City. From kilometer 20 to the end, the Canal runs in a northerly direction. At this point, the Canal is connected with Lake Texcoco, the lowest lake in the Valley, by means of sluices, and passing through Lakes San Cristóbal, Xaltocan and Zumpango, controls the water level of all of them. From kilometer 20 to the junction of the Tunnel, the bottom width is 6.50 meters and with a depth varying between 10 meters and 22 meters. This section is calculated to carry off 18 cubic meters of water per second. The Canal has a total fall of 8.88 meters with uniform side slopes, except in a few places where slips occurred owing to bad ground. The total excavation exceeded 12,000,000 cubic meters, of which 7,200,000 cubic meters were excavated by dredgers and 4,800,000 cubic meters by hand-labor." SMA: PEA, Box 16/3: "Mr. Body's notes," and Mr. J. Body, "The Drainage of the Valley of Mexico," London, 1901.
49 SMA: PEA, Box. 16/3: Mr. J. Body, "The Drainage of the Valley of Mexico," London, 1901.
50 Espinosa and Lombardo, "Reseña técnica de la ejecución," 1: 480–99.
51 Esparza, "Reseña administrativa y económica," 1: 544–45.
52 SMA: PEA, Box 17: "The Drainage System of the Valley of Mexico," by Sr. Don Matías Romero, Mexican Minister at Washington, n.d.
53 Ibid.
54 *La salubridad e higiene pública*, 125.
55 Another type of sewer system was the separate sewer system. Two separate drainage systems were build, one for sewage (a completely sealed network) and the other for rainfall. This system was adopted in London and in other

British cities and in Italy, and it was the commonest system in the United States. See Goubert, *Conquest of Water*, 62–63.
56   AHCM, Policía, Salubridad, Epidemias, vol. 3675, exp. 24.
57   Tomes, *Gospel of Germs*, 8, and Goubert, *Conquest of Water*, 62–63.
58   Ayuntamiento Constitucional de México, *Documentos relativos al drenaje de la ciudad de México* (Mexico City: Tipografía de la Oficina Impresora del Timbre, Palacio Nacional, 1897), 2.
59   Ibid., 3.
60   Ibid., 3.
61   Alan Knight, "Revolutionary Project, Recalcitrant People: Mexico, 1910–1940," in *The Revolutionary Process in Mexico. Essays on Political and Social Change, 1880–1940*, edited by Jaime E. Rodríguez (Los Angeles: UCLA, Latin American Center Publications, 1990), 236–38. On the conflicts between traditional and 'scientific' medical practices in Mexico City during the final decades of the nineteenth century, see Claudia Agostoni, "Médicos científicos y médicos ilícitos en la ciudad de México durante el porfiriato," *Estudios de Historia Moderna y Contemporánea de México* 19 (1999), 13–31.
62   *Memoria del Consejo Superior de Salubridad, 1884–1886. Memoria que el Presidente del Consejo Superior de Salubridad rinde a la Secretaría de Gobernación. De los trabajos ejecutados por ese cuerpo en el periodo transcurrido de noviembre de 1884 á junio de 1886* (Mexico City: Imprenta de Gobierno en el Ex-Arzobispado, 1887), 17.
63   Ayuntamiento Constitucional de México, *Documentos relativos*, 3.
64   Ibid., 6.
65   The use of charcoal and other chemical disinfectants and filters was widely practised in France after the mid-eighteenth century: see Corbin, *Foul and the Fragrant*, 121–27; and Goubert, *Conquest of Water*, 97–98. Their use in Mexico City was examined by Máximo Silva in his book *Higiene popular: Colección de conocimientos y consejos indispensables para evitar las enfermedades y prolongar la vida, arreglada para uso de las familias* (Mexico City: Departamento de Talleres Gráficos, 1917), 577–96.
66   *Boletín del Consejo Superior de Salubridad* 3, no. 3 (30 September 1881): 2. The concern regarding putrefying matter in mid-Victorian cities has been studied by Christopher Hamlin, "Providence and Putrefaction: Victorian Sanitarians and the Natural Theology of Health and Disease," *Victorian Studies* 28, no. 3 (Spring 1985): 381–411.
67   *Boletín del Consejo Superior de Salubridad* 3, no. 3 (30 September 1881): 4.
68   Corbin, *Foul and the Fragrant*, 115–16.
69   López Rosado, *Los servicios públicos de la ciudad de México* (Mexico City: Editorial Porrúa, 1976), 220.
70   SMA: PEA, Box 17: "Report of the Valley Drainage Works and Sanitation Works of Mexico City, 1896."
71   *Informe leído por el C. Presidente de la República al abrirse el tercer periodo de sesiones del XXI Congreso de la Unión* (Mexico City: Tip. y Lit. "La Europea," 1903), 8.
72   Moisés González Navarro, *Población y sociedad en México (1900–1970)* (Mexico City: Universidad Nacional Autónoma de México, 1974), 1: 253.
73   SMA: PEA, Box 17: "The Drainage System of the Valley of Mexico," by Sr. Don Matías Romero, Mexican Minister at Washington, n.d.

74 AHCM, Desagüe, vol. 745, exp. 152.
75 *El Imparcial*, 8 March 1900.
76 Prantl and Groso, *La ciudad de México*, 911.
77 Luis Lara y Pardo, *La prostitución en México* (Mexico City and Paris: Librería de Ch. Bouret, 1908), 108.
78 Ibid., 19.
79 Federico Gamboa, *Santa* (Barcelona: Editorial Araluce, 1903). José Emilio Pacheco has stated that by 1939, the year Gamboa died, *Santa* had already sold more than 60,000 copies, notably becoming the first best-seller in Mexican history; it has been incessantly published since then; it inspired Agustín Lara to compose a song, it became a film in 1918, 1931, 1943 and 1967 and numerous adaptations of the novel have been produced in the theatre and given rise to other films. See José Emilio Pacheco, *Diario de Federico Gamboa (1892–1939)* Prólogo, selección y notas de José Emilio Pacheco (Mexico City: Siglo XXI, 1977), 15–16.
80 Lara y Pardo, *La prostitución*, 54–55.
81 Lara y Pardo quotes Alexandre Parent-Duchâtelet throughout *La prostitución in México*. The appeal of sewers and prostitution during the nineteenth century can be clearly seen in the works of Alexandre Parent-Duchâtelet. See Alexandre Parent-Duchâtelet, *La Prostitution à Paris au XIX siècle*. Texte présenté et annoté par Alain Corbin (Paris: Seuil, 1981). See also Rosalina Estrada Urroz, "Entre la tolerancia y la prohibición de la prostitución. El pensamiento del higienista Parent Duchatelet," in *México – Francia. Memoria de una sensibilidad común, siglos XIX-XX*, coordinated by Javier Pérez Siller (Mexico: Benemérita Universidad Autónoma de Puebla – CEMCA – El Colegio de San Luis, 1998), 307–29.
82 Pacheco, *Diario de Federico Gamboa*, 25–29.
83 Federico Gamboa, *Santa* (Mexico City: Editorial Grijalbo, 1979), 267–68. The original passage quoted is the following: "Santa bajaba, siempre más abajo, siempre más; ... una fuerza sobrehumana la ... [ha] echado a rodar con empuje formidable por todas las lobregueces de las cimas sin fondo de la enorme ciudad corrompida. En ellas rodaba Santa, en los sótanos pestilenciales y negros del vicio inferior, a la manera en que las aguas sucias e impuras de los albañales subterráneos galopan enfurecidas por los oscuros intestinos de las calles, con siniestro glú glú, dc líquido aprisionado que en invariable dirección ha de correr aunque se oponga, aunque se arremoline en ángulos y oquedades sospechosas y hediondas, que los de arriba no conocen ... Allá va el agua, incognoscible, sin cristales en su lomo, sin frescor en sus linfas; conduciendo detritus y microbios, lo que apesta y lo que mata; retratando lo negro, lo escondido, lo innombrable que no debe mostrarse; arrojando por cada respiradero de reja, un vaho pesado, un rumor congojoso y ronco de cansancio, de tristeza, de duelo ... allá va, expulsada de la ciudad y de las gentes, a golpearse contra los hierros de la salida, a morir en el mar, que la amortaja y guarda, que quizá sea el único que recuerde que nació pura; en la montaña, que apagó la sed y fecundó los campos, que fue rocío, perfume, vida."
84 See Frank Mort, *Dangerous Sexualities; Medico-Moral Politics in England since 1830, 2nd ed.* (London and New York: Routledge, 1987), 59–64.
85 A manuscript that explores the figure of the prostitute in Mexican cultural nationalism is "Virgen de Medianoche": La canonización de la prostituta

en el nacionalismo cultural mexicano," by Sergio de la Mora, undated unpublished manuscript. On Porfirian morality and women, see Enriqueta Tuñón Pablos, et al., *El albúm de la mujer. Antología ilustrada de las mexicanas. El Porfiriato y la Revolución*, vol. 4 (Mexico City: Instituto Nacional de Antropología e Historia, 1991); William E. French, "Prostitutes and Guardian Angels: Women, Work and the Family in Porfirian Mexico," *Hispanic American Historical Review* 72, no. 4 (1992): 529–53; Carmen Ramos Escandón, "Señoritas Porfirianas: Mujer e Ideología en el México Progresista, 1880–1910," in *Presencia y transparencia: La mujer en la historia de México*, edited by Carmen Ramos Escandón (Mexico City: El Colegio de México, 1992), 143–61; Verena Radkau, "Imágenes de la mujer en la sociedad porfirista. Viejos mitos en ropaje nuevo," *Revista Encuentro: El Colegio de Jalisco* 4, no. 3 (1987), 5–39, and Radkau, "Hacia la construcción del 'eterno femenino': El discurso científico del Porfiriato al servicio de una sociedad disciplinaria," *Papeles de la Casa Chata* 6, no. 8 (1991), 23–34

86   *El Imparcial*, 16 March 1900.
87   *Diario del Hogar,* 18 March 1900.
88   Esparza, "Reseña administrativa y económica," 1: 634.
89   "Inauguración de las Obras del Desagüe. Datos históricos y crónica de la Fiesta,"*El Imparcial,* 18 March 1900.
90   Ibid.
91   Bazant, "La enseñanza y la práctica," 265.
92   Ibid., 265–66, and Rodney D. Anderson, *Outcasts in Their Own Land. Mexican Industrial Workers, 1906–1911* (Illinois: De Kalb Northern Illinois University Press, 1976), 20.
93   *El Imparcial*, 19 March 1900.
94   Ibid., 22 March 1900.
95   *Diario del Hogar*, 1 April 1900.
96   *El Imparcial*, 15 October 1904.
97   Gilbert M. Joseph and Allen Wells, "Modernizing Visions, *Chilango* Blueprints, and Provincial Growing Pains: Mérida at the Turn of the Century," *Mexican Studies/ Estudios Mexicanos* 8, no. 2 (Summer 1992): 170.
98   Carlos Contreras Cruz, "La ciudad de Puebla en el siglo XIX: espacio y población," in *La ciudad y el campo en la historia de México. Papers presented at the VII Conference of Mexican and the Unites States Historians, Oaxaca – 1985* (Mexico City: Universidad Nacional Autónoma de México, 1992a), 1: 341; and, by the same author, "Ciudad y salud en el Porfiriato. La política urbana y el saneamiento de Puebla (1880–1906)," *Siglo XIX. Cuadernos de Historia* 1, no. 3 (June 1992): 66–68. Also see Eduardo Flores Clair, "Trabajo, salud y muerte: Real del Monte 1874," *Siglo XIX. Cuadernos de Historia* 1, no. 3 (1992): 9–28.
99   Contreras Cruz, "Ciudad y salud en el Porfiriato," 60–61.
100 Ibid., 71–72.
101 Contreras Cruz, "La ciudad de Puebla," 1: 341.
102 In 1877, the exports of henequen amounted to 9,444,282 kilograms; by 1880 they rose to 18,178,994; in 1881 to 24,911,587; by 1883 to 32,651,597, and in 1885 to 43,063,891 kilograms. See Alejandra García Quintanilla, "Salud y progreso en Yucatán en el XIX. Mérida: el sarampión de 1882," *Siglo XIX. Cuadernos de Historia* 1, no. 3 (June 1992): 46.
103 Ibid., 36–44.

104 Joseph and Wells, "Modernizing Visions," 188–89.
105 Ibid., 195.
106 Ibid., 195–200.
107 Ibid., 190.
108 García, *Crónica oficial de las fiestas*, 212–13. See also "Discurso pronunciado por el señor Ingeniero don Norberto Domínguez, Director General de Correos, en el acto de la inauguración de las obras de provisión de aguas potables á la ciudad de México, el 21 de septiembre de 1910," which refers to the conquest of water achieved by the Mexican engineers as comparable only to the achievements of the Roman Empire in ibid., 109–11.
109 García, *Crónica oficial de las fiestas*, "Obras de ensanche del Desagüe del Valle," 215–18. Also see "Discurso pronunciado por el señor Ingeniero don José Ramón de Ibarrola, Director de la Comisión Hidrográfica, en el acto de la inauguración de varias obras del Desagüe del Valle de México, el 26 de septiembre de 1910," 111–14.
110 See the information regarding the Exposición Popular de Higiene in *Crónica oficial de las fiestas*, 261–64, and AHSS. Salubridad Pública. Congresos y Convenciones, cajas 9 y 10. The city also hosted a National Medical Congress where the latest and most important scientific and medical achievements of Mexican physicians and hygienists were discussed.
111 García, *Crónica oficial de las fiestas*, 261.
112 The following were the lectures that took place in the Exhibition of Hygiene in September 1910: 5 September, Dr. Luis E. Ruiz: "Progresos alcanzados en Higiene y Salubridad en la Capital de la República y en el Distrito y Territorios Federales en el siglo que ahora termina." 6 September, Prof. José Donaciano Morales: "Comestibles y Bebidas, expendios de ellas incluyendo los mercados." 9 September, Prof. José de la Luz Gómez: "Matanzas, expendios de carnes, establos y todo lo relativo a Policía sanitaria con relación a animales." 12 September, Dr. Domingo Orvañanos: "Progresos alcanzados en la construcción de habitaciones desde el punto de vista sanitario." 13 September, Dr. Luis E. Ruiz: "Pavimentación de las calles y plazas, riego y barrido de calles desde el principio de la Independencia hasta la fecha." 13 September, engineer Miguel Quevedo: "Espacio libres, sistemas de parques y reservas forestales de las ciudades." 24 September, Dr. Nicolás Ramirez Arellano: "Esfuerzos que se han hecho para combatir las enfermedades transmisibles (tifo, tuberculosis, etc.)." 26 September, engineer Roberto Gayol: "Saneamiento de la Ciudad de México," and engineer Ramón Ibarrola: "Desagüe del Valle de México." 27 September, Dr. Jesús González Ureña: "Progresos alcanzados en la higiene escolar." 28 September, Dr. Eduardo Liceaga: "Progresos realizados en la extinción de las grandes epidemias: Cólera, peste bubónica, fiebre amarilla. Progresos alcanzados en México en lo relativo a Policía Sanitaria Internacional." 29 September, engineer Manuel Marroquin y Rivera: "Provisión de Agua Potable. Obras llevadas a cabo para realizar esta mejora."
113 See *La salubridad é higiene pública en los Estados Unidos Mexicanos. Brevísima reseña de los progresos alcanzados desde 1810 hasta 1910, Publicada por el Consejo Superior de Salubridad, bajo cuyos auspicios tuvo á bien poner la Secretaría de Estado y del Despacho de Gobernación las Conferencias y la Exposición Popular de Higiene, con las cuales se sirvió contribuir a la celebración del Primer Centenario de la Independencia Nacional. Año del Centenario, 1910.* (Mexico City: Casa Metodista de Publicaciones, 1910).

114 "Conferencia del Doctor Eduardo Liceaga titulada: Progresos alcanzados en la higiene de 1810 a la fecha," AHSS, Salubridad Pública. Congresos y Convenciones, exp. 9, caja 9.
115 Ibid.
116 In 1880, the pathogenic organisms of typhoid, leprosy and malaria were identified; in 1882, the disease organism of tuberculosis; in 1883, cholera and streptococcus; in 1884, diphtheria, typhoid, tetanus; in 1894, plague; in 1898, the dysentery bacillus. For a complete account of these events see Rosen, *History of Public Health*, 290–303.
117 AHSS, Salubridad Pública, Congresos y Convenciones, exp. 9, caja 9.
118 On drinking water availability and its distribution in Mexico City from 1870 to 1920, see José Luis Bribiesca Castrejón, *El agua potable en la república mexicana* (Mexico City: Talleres Gráficos de la Nación, 1958), 55–70; Miguel S. Macedo, *Mi barrio (segunda mitad del siglo XIX), Ensayo presentado a la Sociedad de Historia Local de la Ciudad de México en 1927* (Mexico City: editorial 'Cvultura,' 1927), 24–25, 50; Manuel Marroquín y Rivera, *Memoria descriptiva de las obras de provisión de aguas potables para la ciudad de México* (Mexico City: Imprenta y Litografía Müller Hnos, 1914); and Peñafiel, *Memoria sobre las aguas potables*, 49–56.
119 Peñafiel, *Memoria sobre las aguas potables*, 67; and Marroquín y Rivera, *Memoria descriptiva de las obras*, 31–33, 555.
120 Ibid.
121 Ibid.
122 Silva, *Higiene popular*.
123 AHCM, Desagüe, Gobernación, Obras Públicas, vol. 752, exp. 27.
124 Knight, "Revolutionary Project," 243–44.
125 Alvarez Amézquita et al., *Historia de la salubridad*, 2: 44.
126 González Navarro, *Población y sociedad en México*, 1: 229.
127 Alvarez Amézquita et al., *Historia de la salubridad*, 2: 44.
128 Ibid., 97.
129 Bruno Latour, *The Pasteurization of France*, translated by Alan Sheridan and John Low (Cambridge and London: Harvard University Press, 1988), 54–56.
130 Alberto J. Pani, *La higiene en México* (Mexico City: Imprenta de J. Ballescá, 1916). Also see Julio Frenk Mora, "La Salud Pública," in *Contribuciones mexicanas al conocimiento médico*, edited by Hugo Aréchiga and Juan Somolinos Palencia (Mexico City: Fondo de Cultura Económica – Secretaría de Salud, 1993), 577–78.
131 Douglas Wertz Richmond, *Venustiano Carranza's Nationalist Struggle, 1893–1920* (Lincoln: University of Nebraska Press, 1983), 170.
132 Pani, *La higiene en México*, 8.
133 Ibid., 17–19.
134 Ibid., 8.
135 Ibid., 41.
136 Ibid., 35.
137 Ibid., 49.
138 Ibid., 153. Pani may have been acquainted with the novel *Los de Abajo*, written by doctor Mariano Azuela. This novel was first published in 23 instalments during the armed phase of the Revolution in the newspaper *El Paso del Norte* (El Paso, Texas) between October and November 1915. It appeared in book form in December 1915, also in El Paso, Texas, and was

again published in 1917 in Tampico. A different possible source of influence on Pani is the naturalist novel of Federico Gamboa, who, as José Emilio Pacheco has shown, used the phrase "los de abajo" in at least three of his books: *Santa* (1903), *Reconquista* (1908), and *La Llaga* (1913). See Pacheco, *Diario de Federico Gamboa,* 26–27. For a detailed account of Azuela's life and work see Luis Leal, *Mariano Azuela* (New York: Twayne Publishers Inc., 1971) and Charles Griffin, *Azuela. Los de Abajo. Critical Guide to Spanish Texts* (London: Grant & Cutler, 1993).
139 Pani, *La higiene en México,* 191.
140 Alan Knight, "Popular Culture and the Revolutionary State in Mexico, 1910–1940," *Hispanic American Historical Review* 74, no. 3 (1994): 393.
141 Alvarez Amézquita et al., *Historia de la salubridad,* 2: 104–5.
142 González Navarro, *Población y sociedad en México,* 1: 394–98.
143 Abel, *Health, Hygiene and Sanitaion,* 6, 8.

Notes to Epilogue

1 Marshall Berman, *All That Is Solid Melts Into Air: The Experience of Modernity* (London: Verso, 1990), 242.
2 Márquez Morfín, *La desigualdad ante la muerte,* 148.
3 Héctor Aguilar Camín and Lorenzo Meyer, *In the Shadow of the Mexican Revolution: Contemporary Mexican History, 1910–1989,* Translated by Luis Alberto Fierro (Austin: University of Texas Press, 1994), 72–73.
4 See Knight, "Popular Culture," 393.

Bibliography

Archives

AHCM: Archivo Histórico de la Ciudad de México, Mexico City. Fondo Ayuntamiento de la Ciudad de México
Aguas, arquerías y acueductos
Aguas, edificios públicos
Arboledas
Colonias
Consejo Superior de Gobierno del Distrito. Salubridad e higiene
Demarcaciones – cuarteles
Desagüe
Desagüe. Gobernación. Obras públicas
Gobierno del Distrito. Obras públicas
Historia. Inundaciones
Historia. Monumentos
Paseos – Paseo de la Reforma
Policía. Salubridad. Cólera morbus
Policía. Salubridad. Epidemias
Salubridad – Consejo de Salubridad

AHSS: Archivo Histórico de la Secretaría de Salud, Mexico City. Fondo: Salubridad Pública
Congresos y Convenciones
Epidemiología
Higiene Pública
Salubridad en el Distrito Federal

SMA: Library of the Science Museum, London
Records of S. Pearson & Sons

Newspaper Sources and Periodicals

Boletín del Consejo Superior del Distrito Federal
El Diario del Hogar
El Imparcial
El Mundo Ilustrado
El Municipio Libre
El Siglo XIX
El Tiempo
El Universal
La Gaceta Médica de México
La Mujer Mexicana. Revista mensual, científico literaria
La Voz de México

Primary and Secondary Sources

Abel, Christopher. *Health, Hygiene and Sanitation in Latin America c. 1870 to c. 1950.* Institute of Latin American Studies, Research Papers 42. London: University of London, 1996.

Ades, Dawn. *Art in Latin America. The Modern Era, 1820–1980.* London: The Hayward Gallery, 1986.

Agostoni, Claudia. "Médicos científicos y médicos ilícitos en la ciudad de México durante el porfiriato." *Estudios de Historia Moderna y Contemporánea de México* 19 (1999): 13–31.

———. "Sanitation and Public Works in Late Nineteenth Century Mexico City." *Quipu. Revista Latinoamericana de Historia de las Ciencias y la Tecnología* 12, no. 2 (May–August 1999): 187–201.

———. "Salud pública y control social en la ciudad de México a fines del siglo diecinueve." *Historia y grafía* 17 (2001): 73–93.

———. "Mexican Hygienists and the Political and Economic Elite during the Porfirio Díaz regime. The Case of Mexico City (1876–1910)," in *Les Hygiénistes, Enjeux, modèles et pratiques (XVIIIe–XXe siècles)*, sous la direction de Patrice Bourdelais (Paris: Éditions Belin, 2001), 193–210.

———. "Discurso médico, cultura higiénica y la mujer en la ciudad de México al cambio de siglo (XIX-XX)." *Mexican Studies/Estudios Mexicanos* 18, no. 1 (Winter 2002): 1–22.

———. "Las delicias de la limpieza: la higiene en la ciudad de México," in *Bienes y vivencias. El siglo XIX mexicano*, edited and compiled by Anne Staples. In *Historia de la vida cotidiana en México*, coordinated by Pilar Gonzalbo. Mexico City: El Colegio de México – Fondo de Cultura Económica, in press.

Aguilar Camín, Héctor and Lorenzo Meyer. *In the Shadow of the Mexican Revolution. Contemporary Mexican History, 1910–1989.* Translated by Luis Alberto Fierro. Austin: University of Texas Press, 1994.

Alcocer, Alfonso. *La columna de la Independencia.* Mexico City: Ediciones de la Delegación Cuauhtémoc, Departamento del Distrito Federal, n.d.

Alfaro, José. *Higiene pública. Algunas palabras acerca de la influencia higiénica de las arboledas y necesidad de reglamentar su uso entre nosotros.* Prueba escrita para el examen general de medicina, cirugía y obstetricia. Mexico City: Terrazas Impresora, San José de Gracia 5, 1892.

Almanaque Bouret para el año de 1897. Formado bajo la dirección de Raúl Mille y Alberto Leduc. Facsimile edition. Mexico City: Instituto de Investigaciones Dr. José María Luis Mora, 1992.

Alonso, Manuel *Enciclopedia del idioma. Diccionario histórico y moderno de la lengua española (siglos XII al XX)*. Madrid: Aguilar, 1958.

Alva Martínez, Enrique. "La búsqueda de una identidad." In *La arquitectura mexicana del siglo XX*, edited by Fernando González Gortazar. Mexico City: Consejo Nacional para la Cultura y las Artes, 1994.

Alvarez Amézquita, José et al. *Historia de la salubridad y de la asistencia en México*. 4 Vols. Mexico City: Secretaría de Salubridad y Asistencia, 1960.

Anderson, Rodney, D. *Outcasts in Their Own Land: Mexican Industrial Workers, 1906–1911*. Illinois: De Kalb Northern Illinois University Press, 1976.

Armus, Diego. "Tutelaje, higiene y prevención. Una ciudad modelo para la Argentina de comienzos de siglo." In *Medio Ambiente y Urbanización. Homenaje a Jorge E. Hardoy*. Buenos Aires: Instituto Internacional del Medio Ambiente y Desarrollo, IIEDAL, 1993.

Arnáiz y Freg, Arturo and Claude Bataillon, eds. *La intervención francesa y el Imperio de Maximiliano cien años después, 1862–1962*. Mexico City: Asociación Mexicana de Historiadores – Instituto Francés de América Latina, 1965.

Ayuntamiento Constitucional de México. *Documentos relativos al drenaje de la ciudad de México*. Mexico City: Tipografía de la Oficina Impresora del Timbre, Palacio Nacional, 1897.

Báez Macías, Enrique. "Ordenanzas para el establecimiento de alcaldes de barrio en la Nueva España; ciudades de México y de San Luis Potosí." *Boletín del Archivo General de la Nación*, 2a serie, X, 1–2, enero-junio, 1969.

Bancroft, Hubert Howe. *Resources and Developments of Mexico*. San Francisco: The Brancroft Company Publishing, 1893.

Bartra, Roger. "Mexican Oficio: The Miseries and Splendors of Culture." *Third Text* 14 (1991): 7–16.

Bataillon, Claude. *La ciudad y el campo en el México central*. Mexico City: Siglo XXI, 1972.

Bazant, Jan. "From Independence to the Liberal Republic, 1821–1867." In *Mexico Since Independence*, edited by Leslie Bethell. Cambridge: Cambridge University Press, 1991.

Bazant, Mílada. "La enseñanza y la práctica de la ingeniería durante el Porfiriato." *Historia Mexicana* 3 (1984): 254–97.

_____. *Historia de la educación durante el Porfiriato*. Mexico City: El Colegio de México, 1993.

Beecher, Henry C. *A Trip to Mexico*. Toronto: Willing & Williamson, 1880.

Beezley, William. *Judas at the Jockey Club and Other Episodes of Porfirian Mexico*. Lincoln and London: University of Nebraska Press, 1987.

Beezley, William and Judith Ewell, eds. *The Human Tradition in Latin America: The Nineteenth Century*. Wilmington: Scholarly Resources, 1989.

Beezley, William, Cheryl English Martin and William E. French, eds. *Rituals of Rule, Rituals of Resistance: Public Celebrations and Popular Culture in Mexico*. Wilmington: Scholarly Resources, 1994.

Belina, Ladislao de. *Proyecto del desagüe y saneamiento de la ciudad y del Valle de México*. Mexico City: Imprenta de Francisco Díaz de León, 1882.

Benchimol, Jaime Larry. *Pereira Passos: Um Haussmann Tropical: A renova ão urbana da cidade do Rio de Janeiro no início do século XX*. Rio de Janeiro: Biblioteca Carioca, 1990.

Benítez Zenteno, Raul. *Analisis Demográfico de México*. Mexico City: Instituto de Investigaciones Sociales, Universidad Nacional Autónoma de México, 1961.

Benjamin, Thomas and Marcial Ocasio-Meléndez, "Organizing the Memory of Modern Mexico: Porfirian Historiography in Perspective, 1880s-1980s." *Hispanic American Historical Review* 62, no. 2 (1984): 323–64.

Berman, Marshall. *All That Is Solid Melts Into Air: The Experience of Modernity*. London: Verso, 1990.

Boret Correa, Antonio. "La arquitectura de la época Porfiriana en México." *Anales de la Universidad de Murcia* 24 (1965–66): 249–309.

Brading, David. "The City in Bourbon Spanish America: Elite and Masses." *Comparative Urban Research* 8, no. 1 (1980): 71–85.

———. *The Origins of Mexican Nationalism*. Cambridge: Centre of Latin American Studies, 1985.

———. "Bourbon Spain and its American Empire." In *Colonial Spanish America*, edited by Leslie Bethell. Cambridge: Cambridge University Press, 1987.

Breña, Juan. "Sobre algunas prácticas religiosas que deben abolirse en beneficio de la higiene." In *Memoria General del IV Congreso Médico Nacional Mexicano efectuado en la ciudad de México del 9 al 25 de septiembre de 1910* (año del Centenario). Mexico City: Tipografía Económica, 1910, 674–81.

Bribiesca Castrejón, José Luis. *El agua potable en la república mexicana*. Mexico City: Talleres Gráficos de la Nación, 1958.

Brief Sketch of the Drainage Works of the Valley of Mexico. Written expressively for the delegates of the Pan-American Congress. Mexico City: Tipografía de Francisco Díaz de León, 1901.

Brown, Jonathan. "Foreign and Native-Born Workers in Porfirian México." *American Historical Review* 98, no. 3 (1993): 786–818.

Browne, E. J., William F. Bynum and Roy Porter. *Dictionary of the History of Science*. London: Macmillan Press, 1983.

Buffington, Robert. *Criminal and Citizen in Modern Mexico*. Lincoln: University of Nebraska Press, 1999.

Bulnes, Francisco. *El desagüe del Valle de México a la luz de la higiene*. Mexico City: Oficina Impresora de Estamillas, Tipografía Palacio Nacional, 1892.

Bustamante, Miguel E. "La situación epidemiológica de México en el siglo XIX." In *Ensayos sobre la historia de las epidemias en México*, edited by Enrique Florescano and Elsa Malvido. Vol. 2. Mexico City: Instituto Mexicano del Seguro Social – Colección Salud y Seguridad Social, Serie Historia, 1982.

Bynum, William F. *Science and the Practice of Medicine in the Nineteenth Century*. London: Routledge, 1994.

Calderón de la Barca, Frances. *Life in Mexico*. Introduction by Manuel Romero de Terreros. London: J.M. Dent & Sons, Ltd, 1954.

Campbells, Reau. *Campbell's New Revised Complete Guide and Descriptive Book of Mexico*. Chicago: Roger & Smith Co, 1909.

Carmagnani, Marcelo. "Territorios, provincias y estados: las transformaciones de los espacios políticos en México, 1750–1850." In *La fundación del Estado mexicano, 1821–1855*, coordinated by Josefina Zoraida Vázquez. Mexico City: Nueva Imagen, 1994.

Carvalho, Paulo Morgan Simoes de. "El azote que hoy nos amaga: cholera, reaction and insurrection in Mexico, 1833." M.A. diss., San José State University, 1996.

Casanova, Rosa and Olivier Debroise. *Sobre la superficie bruñida de un espejo*. Mexico City: Fondo de Cultura Económica, 1989.
Catálogo del Archivo Histórico del Ex Ayuntamiento de la Ciudad de México, 1524–1928. Mexico City: Secretaría de Desarrollo Social, Departamento del Distrito Federal, 1988.
Chalhoub, Sideny. "The Politics of Disease Control: Yellow Fever and Race in Nineteenth Century Rio de Janeiro." *Journal of Latin American Studies* 25: 441–63.
Cházaro García, Laura. "Medir y valorar los cuerpos de una nación: un ensayo sobre la estadística médica del siglo XIX mexicano." Ph.D. diss., Facultad de Filosofía y Letras, Universidad Nacional Autónoma de México, 2000.
Choay, Fran oise. *The Modern City: Planning in the 19th Century*. New York: George Braziller, 1969.
Cipolla, Carlo. *Miasmas and Disease: Public Health and the Environment in the pre-industrial Age*. New Haven: Yale University Press, 1992.
Clement, Jean-Pierre. "El nacimiento de la higiene urbana en la América española del siglo XVIII." *Revista de Indias* 171 (January–June 1983): 77–95.
Coatsworth, John H. *El impacto económico de los ferrocarriles en el Porfiriato: Crecimiento contra desarrollo*. Mexico City: Ediciones Era, 1976.
Código Sanitario de los Estados Unidos Mexicanos. Mexico City: Imprenta del Gobierno Federal en el ex Arzobispado, 1891.
Compendio de providencias de policía de México del Segundo Conde de Revillagigedo. Versión paleográfica, introducción y notas por Ignacio González-Polo. Suplemento al Boletín del Instituto de Investigaciones Bibliográficas, 14. Mexico City: Universidad Nacional Autónoma de México, 1983.
Concise Medical Dictionary Oxford Reference. Oxford: Oxford University Press, 1994.
Condorcet, Jean-Antoine-Nicolas de Caritat, Marquis de. *Esquisse d'un tableau historique des progrès de l'esprit humain*; introduction et notes par Monique et Fran ois Hincker. Paris: Editions Sociales, 1966.
Connolly, Priscilla. *El contratista de Don Porfirio: Obras públicas, deuda y desarrollo desigual*. Mexico City: Fondo de Cultura Económica, 1997.
Contreras Cruz, Carlos. "Ciudad y salud en el Porfiriato: La política urbana y el saneamiento de Puebla (1880–1906)." *Siglo XIX. Cuadernos de Historia* 1, no. 3 (June 1992): 55–76.
_____. "La ciudad de Puebla en el siglo XIX: espacio y población." In *La ciudad y el campo en la historia de México*. Papers presented at the VII Conference of Mexican and the Unites States Historians, Oaxaca – 1985. Vol. 1. Mexico City: Universidad Nacional Autónoma de México, 1992a.
Cooper, Donald. *Epidemic Disease in Mexico City, 1761–1813. An Administrative, Social and Medical Study*. Institute of Latin American Studies. Austin: University of Texas Press, 1965.
Corbin, Alain. *The Foul and the Fragrant. Odour and the French Social Imagination*. Preface by Roy Porter. London: Picador, 1994.
Corominas, Juan. *Diccionario crítico etimológico de la lengua castellana*. Berna: Editorial Francke, 1954.
_____. *Breve diccionario etimológico de la lengua castellana*. Tercera edición muy revisada y mejorada. Madrid: Editorial Gredos, 1973.
Cosio Villegas, Daniel, ed. *Historia moderna de México. La vida política interior. El Porfiriato*. Primera parte. Mexico City: Editorial Hermes, 1970.

Cuadro Geográfico, estadístico, descriptivo e histórico de los Estados Unidos Mexicanos. Mexico City: Oficina Tipográfica de la Secretaría de Fomento, 1885.

Cuenca, Laura M. "Las necesidades de México. México necesita aseo." *La mujer mexicana. Revista mensual, científico literaria* 2, no. 4 (1905): 1–2

Cuenya, Miguel Angel et al. *El cólera de 1833: una nueva patología en México. Causas y efectos.* Mexico City: Instituto Nacional de Antropología e Historia, Colección Divulgación, 1992.

Cueto, Marcos, ed. *Salud, cultura y sociedad en América Latina.* Lima: IEP – Organización Panamericana de la Salud, 1996.

Dávalos, Marcela. *De basura, inmundicias y movimiento o de cómo se limpiaba la ciudad de México a finales del XVIII.* Mexico City: Cienfuegos, 1989.

_____. "La salud, el agua y los habitantes de la ciudad de México. Fines del siglo XVIII y principios del XIX." In *La ciudad de México en la primera mitad del siglo XIX*, comp. Regina Hernández Franyuti. Vol. 1. Mexico City: Instituto de Investigaciones Dr. José María Luis Mora, 1994.

De la Fuente, Manuel. *Estudio sobre las aplicaciones de la higiene contra la invasión del cólera epidémico.* Presentado en el examen de medicina y cirugía. Mexico City: Oficina Tipográfica de la Secretaría de Fomento, 1885.

De la Mora, Sergio. "*Virgen de Medianoche: La canonización de la prostituta en el nacionalismo cultural mexicano.*" Undated unpublished manuscript.

De la Peña, Sergio and James W. Wilkie. *La estadística económica en Mexico: Los orígenes.* Mexico City: Siglo XXI, 1994.

Delaporte, Fran ois. *Disease and Civilization: The Cholera in Paris.* Cambridge: MIT Press, 1986.

Díaz-Trechuelo Spínola, María de Lourdes et al. "El Virrey Don Juan Vicente de Güemez Pacheco, Segundo Conde de Revillagigedo (1789–1794)." In *Virreyes de Nueva España en el reinado de Carlos IV.* Dirección y estudio preliminar de José Antonio Calderón Quijano. Vol. 1. Sevilla: Escuela de Estudios Hispanoamericanos, 1972.

Díaz y de Ovando, Clementina. "La ciudad de México en 1904." *Historia Mexicana* 24 (1974): 122–44.

_____. Foreword to *Vicente Riva Palacio. Cuentos del General.* Mexico City: Editorial Porrúa, 1986.

_____. *Las fiestas patrias en el México de hace un siglo, 1883.* Mexico City: Centro de Estudios de Historia de México, 1983.

Diccionario Porrúa de historia, biografía y geografía de México. Mexico City: Editorial Porrúa, 1976.

Diccionario Porrúa de historia, biografía y geografía de México. Quinta edición, corregida y aumentada con un suplemento. Mexico City: Editorial Porrúa, 1986.

Dictamen que presenta la comisión nombrada por la Junta General del Ramo de Pulques al Señor Gobernador del Distrito impugnando el vulgar error de que el consumo de esta bebida nacional es causa de criminalidad en México. Mexico City: Talleres de la Tipografía Artística, 1896.

"Discurso sobre la policía de México." *Reflexiones y apuntes sobre la ciudad de México (fines de la Colonia).* Versión paleográfica, introducción y notas por Ignacio González-Polo. Colección Distrito Federal 4. Mexico City: Departamento del Distrito Federal, 1984.

Dollero, Adolfo. *México al día (Impresiones y notas de un viaje).* Mexico City: Librería V. de C. Bouret, 1911.

Douglas, Mary. *Purity and Danger: An Analysis of the Concepts of Pollution and Taboo*. London: Routledge, 1994.
Drewes, Michael. "Proyecto de remodelación del Palacio de Chapultepec en la época del Emperador Maximiliano." *Anales del Instituto de Investigaciones Estéticas* 51 (1983): 73–82.
Dublán, Manuel and José María Lozano. *Legislación mexicana o colección completa de las disposiciones legislativas expedidas desde la Independencia de la República*. Vols. 2, 12, 13, 17. Mexico City: Imprenta de Eduardo Dublán, 1876–1887.
Duffy, John. *The Sanitarians: A History of American Public Health*. Urbana: University of Illinois Press, 1990.
Durand Ponte, Victor Manuel. *México: La formación de un país dependiente*. Mexico City: Instituto de Investigaciones Sociales – Universidad Nacional Aautónoma de México, 1979.
Eder, Rita. "The Icons of Power and Popular Art." In *Mexican Monuments, Strange Encounters*, edited by Helen Escobedo. New York: Abbeville Press, 1989.
Eder, Eder, "La fotografía en México en el siglo XIX." *Historia del arte mexicano*. Vol. 9. Mexico City: Secretaría de Educación Pública – Instituto Nacional de Bellas Artes – Salvat, 1982.
Eguiarte Sakar, María Estela. "Los jardines en México y la idea de ciudad decimonónica." *Historias 27*. Revista de la Dirección de Estudios Históricos del Instituto Nacional de Antropología e Historia (October 1991-March 1992): 129–38.
Epstein, Isidro. *La mortalidad en México*. Mexico City: Sociedad Mexicana de Geografía y Estadística, 1894.
Escobedo, Helen, ed. "Foreword" to *Mexican Monuments, Strange Encounters*. New York: Abbeville Press, 1989.
Espantoso Rodríguez, María Teresa et al. "Imágenes para la Nación Argentina. Conformación de un eje monumental urbano en Buenos Aires entre 1811 y 1910." In *Arte, Historia e Identidad en América: Visiones Comparativas. XVII Coloquio Internacional de Historia del Arte*. Vol. 2. Mexico City: Instituto de Investigaciones Estéticas, Universidad Nacional Autónoma de México, 1994.
Esparza, Rosendo. "Reseña administrativa y económica de la Junta Directiva del Desagüe del valle de México, 1886–1900." In *Memoria histórica, técnica y administrativa de las Obras del Desagüe del Valle de México. 1449–1900, publicada por orden de la Junta Directiva del mismo Desagüe*. Vol. 1. Mexico City: Tipografía de la Oficina Impresora de Estampillas, Palacio Nacional, 1902.
Espinosa, Luis. "Reseña histórica y técnica de las obras del desagüe del valle de México. 1856–1900." In *Memoria histórica, técnica y administrativa de las Obras del Desagüe del Valle de México. 1449–1900, publicada por orden de la Junta Directiva del mismo Desagüe*. Vol. 1. Mexico City: Tipografía de la Oficina Impresora de Estampillas, Palacio Nacional, 1902.
Espinosa, Luis and Isidro Díaz Lombardo. "Reseña técnica de la ejecución del Gran Canal, y de las obras de arte. 1886–1900." In *Memoria histórica, técnica y administrativa de las Obras del Desagüe del Valle de México. 1449–1900, publicada por orden de la Junta Directiva del mismo Desagüe*. Vol. 1. Mexico City: Tipografía de la Oficina Impresora de Estampillas, Palacio Nacional, 1902.
Estadísticas sociales del porfiriato, 1877–1910. Mexico City: Talleres Gráficos de la Nación, 1956.

Estrada Urroz, Rosalina. "Entre la tolerancia y la prohibición de la prostitución. El pensamiento del higienista Parent Duchatelet." In *México – Francia. Memoria de una sensibilidad común, siglos XIX-XX*, coordinated by Javier Pérez Siller. Mexico: Benemérita Universidad Autónoma de Puebla – CEMCA – El Colegio de San Luis, 1998.

Estudios referentes a la desecación del lago de Texcoco año de 1895. Mexico City: Oficina Tipográfica de la Secretaría de Fomento, 1895.

Evans, Richard J. *Death in Hamburg: Society and Politics in the Cholera Years, 1830–1910.* Oxford: Clarendon Press, 1987.

Fernández, Justino. *El arte del siglo XIX en México.* Mexico City: Imprenta Universitaria, 1967.

Fernández Christlieb, Federico. "La influencia francesa en el urbanismo de la ciudad de México: 1775–1910." In *México – Francia. Memoria de una sensibilidad común, siglos XVIII-XX*, coordinated by Javier Pérez Siller. Mexico: Benemérita Universidad Autónoma de Puebla – El Colegio de San Luis A.C. – CEMCA, 1998.

Figueroa Domenech, J. *Guía general descriptiva de la República Mexicana.* 2 Vols. Mexico City: Araluce, 1889.

Flandrau, Charles. *Viva Mexico! A Traveller's Account of Life in Mexico.* London: Eland, 1990.

Florescano, Enrique and Elsa Malvido, eds. *Ensayo sobre la historia de las epidemias en México.* Vol. 2. Mexico City: Colección Salud y Seguridad Social – Serie Historia, Instituto Mexicano del Seguro Social, 1982.

Flores Clair, Eduardo. "Trabajo, salud y muerte: Real del Monte 1874." *Siglo XIX. Cuadernos de Historia* 1, no. 3 (1992): 9–28.

Foucault, Michel. *The Birth of the Clinic: An Archaeology of Medical Perception.* London: Routledge, 1991.

French, William E. "Prostitutes and Guardian Angels: Women, Work and the Family in Porfirian Mexico." *Hispanic American Historical Review* 72, no. 4 (1992): 529–53.

Frenk Mora, José et al. "La Salud Pública." In *Contribuciones mexicanas al conocimiento médico*, edited by Hugo Aréchiga and Juan Somolinos Palencia. Mexico City: Fondo de Cultura Económica – Secretaría de Salud, 1993.

Gamboa, Federico. *Santa.* Mexico City: Editorial Grijalbo, 1979.

García Canclini, Nestor. "México 2000: ciudad sin mapa. Desurbanización, patrimonio y cultura electrónica." *Medio Ambiente y Urbanización: La Ciudad Latinoamericana del Futuro* 10, nos. 43–44 (1993): 111–24.

García Cubas, Antonio. *Atlas geográfico y estadístico de los Estados Unidos Mexicanos.* Mexico City: Oficina Tipográfica de la Secretaría de Fomento, 1884.

———. *Geografía e historia del Distrito Federal.* Facsimile of the 1894 edition. Mexico City: Instituto de Investigaciones Dr. José María Luis Mora, 1993.

García, Genaro. *Crónica Oficial de las Fiestas del Primer Centenario de la Independencia de México.* Mexico City: Talleres del Museo Nacional, 1911. Facsimile edition, Centro de Estudios de Historia de México, 1991.

García Quintana, Josefina. *Cuauhtémoc en el siglo XIX.* Mexico City: Instituto de Investigaciones Históricas – Universidad Nacional Autónoma de México, 1977.

García Quintanilla, Alejandra. "Salud y progreso en Yucatán en el XIX. Mérida: el sarampión de 1882." *Siglo XIX. Cuadernos de Historia* 1, no. 3 (June 1992): 29–54.

Garner, Paul. "The Politics of National Development in Late Porfirian Mexico: the Reconstruction of the Tehuantepec National Railway 1896–1907." *Bulletin of Latin American Research* 14, no. 3 (1995): 339–56.

Garza, Gustavo. "El sistema ferroviario y eléctrico como génesis de la concentración industrial en la ciudad de México (1876–1910)." In *La ciudad y el campo en la historia de México. Papers presented at the VII Conference of Mexican and the Unites States Historians, Oaxaca, 1985*. Vol. 1. Mexico City: Universidad Nacional Autónoma de México, 1992.

Gibson, Charles. *The Aztecs Under Spanish Rule. A History of the Indians of the Valley of Mexico, 1519–1810*. Stanford California: Stanford University Press, 1964.

Gomez Mayorga, Mauricio. "La influencia francesa en la arquitectura y el urbanismo en México." In *La intervención francesa y el Imperio de Maximiliano cien años después, 1862–1962*, edited by Arturo Arnáiz y Freg and Claude Bataillon. Mexico City: Asociación Mexicana de Historiadores – Instituto Francés de América Latina, 1965.

González Navarro, Moisés. "México en una laguna." *Historia Mexicana* 4 (1955): 506–22.

_____. *Historia moderna de Mexico. El porfiriato. La vida social*. Mexico City: Editorial Hermes, 1957.

_____. *Población y sociedad en México (1900–1970)*. 2 vols. Mexico City: Universidad Nacional Autónoma de México, 1974.

González Obregón, Luis. "Reseña histórica del desagüe del Valle de México, 1449–1855." In *Memoria histórica, técnica y administrativa de las Obras del Desagüe del Valle de México. 1449–1900, publicada por orden de la Junta Directiva del mismo Desagüe*. Vol. 1. Mexico City: Tipografía de la Oficina Impresora de Estampillas, Palacio Nacional, 1902.

_____. *Cuauhtémoc. El rey heroico de los mexicanos*. Mexico City: Biblioteca Mínima Mexicana, Libro-Mex Editores, 1955.

_____. *Las calles de México*. Mexico City: Clásicos Mexicanos, Alianza Editorial, 1992.

González-Polo, Ignacio. "La ciudad de México a fines del siglo XVIII- Disquisiciones sobre un manuscrito anónimo." *Historia Mexicana* 101 (1976): 29–47.

Gooch Chambers, Fanny. *Face to Face with the Mexicans*. New York: Howard and Hulbert, 1887.

Gortari, Hira de. "¿Un modelo de urbanización? La ciudad de México a finales del siglo XIX." *Secuencia* 8. Revista Americana de Ciencias Sociales (January–April 1987): 42–52.

_____. "Las ciudades decimonónicas mexicanas: itinerario de estudio." *Colloque: Le Mexique en France. L'Ordinaire Latino-Americain*. 160–61, vol. 2 (novembre 1995–février 1996): 35–42.

Gortari, Hira de and Regina Hernández Franyuti. *La Ciudad de México y el Distrito Federal. Una historia compartida*. Mexico City: Instituto de Investigaciones Dr. José María Luis Mora – Departamento del Distrito Federal, 1988.

_____. *Memoria y Encuentros. La Ciudad de México y el Distrito Federal (1824–1928)*. Mexico City: Instituto de Investigaciones Dr. José María Luis Mora – Departamento del Distrito Federal, 1988a.

Gostkowski, Gustave Baron. *De Paris à Mexico par les Etats-Unis*. Paris: P.V. Stock, 1899.
Goubert, Jean-Pierre. *The Conquest of Water: The Advent of Health in the Industrial Age*. Introduction by Emmanuel Le Roy Ladurie, London: Polity Press, 1986.
Greenhalgh, Paul. *Ephemeral Vistas: The Expositions Universelles, Great Exhibitions and World's Fairs, 1851–1939*. Manchester: Manchester University Press, 1988.
Griffin, Charles. *Azuela. Los de Abajo. Critical Guide to Spanish Texts*. London: Grant and Cutler, 1993.
Guerrero, Julio. *La génesis del crimen en México: Estudio de psiquiatría social*. Mexico City and Paris: Librería de la Viuda de Charles Bouret, 1901.
Güijosa, José. *El Valle de México: Ventajas que resultarán a la salud pública con el desagüe*. Tesis para el examen general de medicina, cirugía y obstetricia. Escuela Nacional de Medicina. Mexico City: Imprenta de Joaquín G. Campos y Comp, 1892.
Gurría Lacroix, Jorge. *El desagüe del valle de México durante la época novohispana*. Mexico City: Universidad Nacional Autónoma de México, 1978.
Gutiérrez Nájera, Manuel. *Escritos inéditos de sabor satírico "Platos del día."* Columbia, Missouri: University of Missouri Press, 1972.
Hale, Charles. "Political and Social Ideas." In *Latin America. Economy and Society, 1870–1930*, edited by Leslie Bethell. Cambridge: Cambridge University Press, 1984.
_____. *The Transformation of Liberalism in Late-Nineteenth Century Mexico*. Princeton, NJ: Princeton University Press, 1989.
Hamlin, Christopher. *A Science of Impurity: Water Analysis in Nineteenth-Century Britain*. Berkeley: University of California Press, 1990.
Hamlin, Christopher. "Providence and Putrefaction: Victorian Sanitarians and the Natural Theology of Health and Disease." *Victorian Studies* 28, no. 3 (Spring 1985), 381–411.
Hannaway, Caroline. "Environment and miasmata." In *Companion Encyclopedia of the History of Medicine*, edited by William F. Bynum and Roy Porter. Vol. 1. London: Routledge, 1993.
Hardoy, Jorge Eduardo. "Theory and Practice of Urban Planning in Europe, 1850–1930: Its Transfer to Latin America." In *Rethinking the Latin American City*, edited by Richard M. Morse and Jorge E. Hardoy. Baltimore: Johns Hopkins University Press, 1992.
Hernández, Vicente Martín. *Arquitectura doméstica de la ciudad de México, 1890–1925*. Mexico City: Escuela de Arquitectura, Universidad Nacional Autónoma de México, 1981.
Hoberman, Louisa. "Bureaucracy and Disaster: Mexico City and the Flood of 1629." *Journal of Latin American Studies* 6 (1974): 211–30.
Hobsbawm, Eric. *The Age of Empire, 1875–1914*. London: Abacus, 1995.
_____ and Terrence Ranger, eds. *The Invention of Tradition*. London: Canto, 1995a.
Howard-Jones, Norman. *The Scientific Background of the International Sanitary Conferences, 1851–1938*. Geneva: World Health Organization, 1975.
Humboldt, Alejandro de. *Ensayo político sobre el reino de la Nueva España*. Estudio preliminar, revisión del texto, notas y anexos de Juan A. Ortega y Medina. Mexico City: Editorial Porrúa, 1966.
Hutchinson, Charles A. "El cólera de 1833: el Día del Juicio en México." *Paginas de los Trabajadores del Estado*, Mexico City (March 1984): 14–26

Informe leído por el C. Presidente de la República al abrirse el tercer periodo de sesiones del XXI Congreso de la Unión. Mexico City: Tip. y Lit. "La Europea," 1903.

Janson, Horst Woldemar. *Nineteenth-Century Sculpture*. London: Thames & Hudson, 1985.

Jiménez Muñoz, Jorge. *La traza del poder: historia de la política y los negocios urbanos en el Distrito Federal, de sus orígenes a la desaparición del ayuntamiento, 1824–1928*. Mexico City: Codex Editores, 1993.

Jones, Gareth A. "The Latin American City as a Contested Space: a Manifesto." *Bulletin of Latin American Research* 13, no. 1 (1994): 1–12.

⸺ and Anne Varley. "The Contest of the City Centre: Street Traders versus Buildings." *Bulletin of Latin American Research* 13, no. 1 (1994): 27–44.

Joseph, Gilbert M., and Allen Wells. "Modernizing Visions, *Chilango* Blueprints, and Provincial Growing Pains: Mérida at the Turn of the Century." *Mexican Studies / Estudios Mexicanos* 8, no. 2 (Summer 1992): 167–215.

Kandell, Jonathan. *La Capital: The Biography of Mexico City*. New York: Random House, 1988.

Katzman, Israel. *Arquitectura del siglo XIX en México*. Mexico City: Trillas, 1988.

Kay Vaughman, Mary. *The State, Education and Social Class in Mexico, 1880–1928*. De Kalb: Northern Illinois University Press, 1982.

Knight, Alan. "Revolutionary Project, Recalcitrant People: Mexico, 1910–1940." In *The Revolutionary Process in Mexico. Essays on Political and Social Change, 1880–1940*, edited by Jaime E. Rodríguez. Los Angeles: UCLA, Latin American Center Publications, 1990.

⸺. "Popular Culture and the Revolutionary State in Mexico, 1910–1940." *Hispanic American Historical Review* 74, no. 3 (1994): 393–444.

La Berge, Ann F. *Mission and Method: The Early-Nineteenth-Century French Public Health Movement*. Cambridge: Cambridge University Press, 1992.

La salubridad é higiene pública en los Estados Unidos Mexicanos. Brevísima reseña de los progresos alcanzados desde 1810 hasta 1910. Publicada por el Consejo Superior de Salubridad, bajo cuyos auspicios tuvo á bien poner la Secretaría de Estado y del Despacho de Gobernación las Conferencias y la Exposición Popular de Higiene, con las cuales se sirvió contribuir a la celebración del Primer Centenario de la Independencia Nacional. Año del Centenario, 1910. Mexico City: Casa Metodista de Publicaciones, 1910.

Lara y Pardo, Luis. *La prostitución en México*. Mexico City and Paris: Librería de Ch. Bouret, 1908.

Latour, Bruno. *The Pasteurization of France*. Translated by Alan Sheridan and John Low. Cambridge and London: Harvard University Press, 1988

Lavedán, Pierre. *Histoire de l'urbanisme. Epoque contemporaine*. Vol. 3. Paris: Henri Laurens, 1952.

Lawrence, Christopher. *Medicine in the Making of Modern Britain, 1700–1920*. London: Routledge, 1994.

Le Goff, Jacques and Jean-Charles Sournia, eds. *Les maladies ont une histoire*. Paris: L'Histoire Seuil, 1985.

Le Roy Ladurie, Emmanuel. "De l'esthétique à la pathologie." In *Histoire de la France urbaine. Sous la direction de Georges Duby. La Ville Classique de la Renaissance aux Revolutions*, edited by Roger Chartier et al. Vol. 3. Paris: Seuil, 1981.

Leal, Luis. *Mariano Azuela*. New York: Twayne Publishers Inc., 1971.

Lemoine Villicaña, Ernesto. *El desagüe del Valle de México durante la época Independiente*. Mexico City: Instituto de Investigaciones Históricas – Universidad Nacional Autónoma de México, 1978.

Levine, Robert. "Images of Progress in Nineteenth-Century Latin America." *Journal of Urban History* 15, no. 3 (May 1989): 304–23.

Lira, Andrés. *Comunidades indígenas frente a la ciudad de México. Tenochtitlán y Tlatelolco, sus pueblos y barrios, 1812–1919*. Mexico City: El Colegio de México – El Colegio de Michoacán, 1983.

——. "Legalización del espacio: la ciudad de México y Distrito Federal, 1874–1884." In *Construcción de la legitimidad política en México*, coordinated by Brian Connaughton, Carlos Illades and Sonia Pérez Toledo. Mexico: El Colegio de Michoacán – Universidad Autónoma Metropolitana – Universidad Nacional Autónoma de México – El Colegio de México, 1999.

Lobato, José Guadalupe. "Higiene pública. Los arbolados, los bosques montañosos y los planos, los jardines, las huertas y los sembrados en las comarcas gerográficas intercontinentales." *Gaceta Médica de México* 16, no. 15 (1 August 1881): 249–59, 274–82.

Lloyd, Geoffrey Ernest Richard, ed. *Hippocratic Writings*. London: Penguin, 1983.

Lombardo de Ruiz, Sonia. "Ideas y proyectos urbanísticos de la ciudad de México, 1788–1850." In *Ciudad de México. Ensayo de construcción de una historia*, edited by Alejandra Moreno Toscano. Mexico City: Instituto Nacional de Antropología e Historia – Seminario de Historia Urbana, Colección Científica 61, 1978.

——, ed. *Antología de textos sobre la ciudad de México en el período de la Ilustración (1788–1792)*. Mexico City: Instituto Nacional de Antropología e Historia, Colección Científica 113, 1982.

——. *El pasado prehispánico en la cultura nacional (Memoria hemerográfica, 1877–1911). El Monitor Republicano (1877–1896)*. Vol. 1. Mexico City: Instituto Nacional de Antropología e Historia – Antologías Serie Historia., 1994.

López Monjardín, Alejandra. *Hacia la ciudad capital: México, 1790–1870*. Mexico City: Dirección de Estudios Históricos – Instituto Nacional de Antropología e Historia, 1985.

López Rosado, Diego. *Historia y pensamiento económico en México. Finanzas públicas – obras públicas*. Mexico City: Universidad Nacional Autónoma de México, 1972.

——. *Los servicios públicos de la ciudad de México*. Mexico City: Editorial Porrúa, 1976.

Los Estados Unidos Mexicanos: Sus progresos en veinte años de paz, 1877–1897. New York: H. A. Rost & Co., 1899.

Luckin, Bill. *Pollution and Control: A Social History of the Thames in the Nineteenth Century*. Bristol: Adam Hilger, 1986.

Macedo, Miguel S. *Mi barrio (segunda mitad del siglo XIX). Ensayo presentado a la Sociedad de Historia Local de la Ciudad de México en 1927*. Mexico City: Editorial 'Cvultura', 1927.

Maldonado, Celia. "El control de las epidemias: modificaciones en la estructura urbana." In *Ciudad de México. Ensayo de construcción de una historia*, edited by Alejandra Moreno Toscano. Mexico City: Instituto Nacional de Antropología e Historia, 1976.

Márquez Morfín, Lourdes. *La desigualdad ante la muerte en la ciudad de México. El tifo y el cólera. (1813 y 1833)*. Mexico City: Siglo XXI, 1994.

Marroquín y Rivera, Manuel. *Memoria descriptiva de las obras de provisión de aguas potables para la ciudad de México*. Mexico City: Imprenta y Litografía Müller Hnos, 1914.

Martínez Cortés, Fernando. *De los miasmas y efluvios al descubrimiento de las bacterias patógenas. Los primeros cincuenta años del Consejo Superior de Salubridad*. Mexico City: Bristol-Myers Squibb de México, 1993.

Mathes, Michael W. "To save a city: the desagüe of Mexico-Huehuetoca, 1607." *The Americas* 26 (1970): 419–38

Maza, Francisco de la. *La ciudad de México en el siglo XVII*. Mexico City: Fondo de Cultura Económica, 1968.

———. *Enrico Martínez, cosmógrafo e impresor de la Nueva España*. Mexico City: Sociedad Mexicana de Geografía y Estadística, 1943.

Meade, Teresa. "'Civilising Rio de Janeiro': The Public Health Campaign and the Riot of 1904." *Journal of Social History* 20, no. 2 (1987): 301–22.

———. "Living Worse and Costing More: Resistance and Riot in Rio de Janeiro." *Journal of Latin American Studies* 21 (1989): 241–66.

Melosi, Martin V., ed. *Pollution and Reform in American Cities, 1870–1930*. Austin and London: University of Texas Press, 1980.

Memoria de las obras del sistema del drenaje profundo del Distrito Federal. 3 vols. Mexico City: Departamento del Distrito Federal, 1975.

Memoria del Consejo Superior de Salubridad, 1884–1886. Memoria que el Presidente del Consejo Superior de Salubridad rinde a la Secretaría de Gobernación. De los trabajos ejecutados por ese cuerpo en el periodo transcurrido de noviembre de 1884 á junio de 1886. Mexico City: Imprenta de Gobierno en el Ex-Arzobispado, 1887.

Memoria del Consejo Superior de Salubridad, 1901. Memoria de los trabajos ejecutados por el Consejo Superior de Salubridad en el año de 1901. Mexico City: Imprenta de Eduardo Dublán, 1902.

Memoria del Consejo Superior de Salubridad, 1905. Memoria de los trabajos ejecutados por el Consejo Superior de Salubridad en el año de 1905. Presentada por el Dr. E. Liceaga, Presidente del Consejo Superior de Salubridad al Secretario de Gobernación. Mexico City: A. Carranza y Compañía Impresores, 1905.

Memoria histórica, técnica y administrativa de las Obras del Desagüe del Valle de México. 1449–1900, publicada por orden de la Junta Directiva del mismo Desagüe. 2 vols. Mexico City: Tipografía de la Oficina Impresora de Estampillas, Palacio Nacional, 1902.

McClary, Andrew. "Germs are Everywhere: The Germ Threat as Seen in Magazine Articles, 1890–1920." *Journal of American Culture* 3, nos. 1–2 (1980): 33–46.

Molina del Villar, Amércia. *Por voluntad divina: escasez, epidemias y otras calamidades en la ciudad de México, 1700–1762*. Mexico City: CIESAS, 1996.

Monnet, Jerôme. "¿Poesía o urbanismo? Utopías urbanas y crónicas de la ciudad de México. (Siglos XVI a XX)." *Historia Mexicana* 39, no. 3 (1990): 727–66.

Monsiváis, Carlos. "La aparición del subsuelo. Sobre la cultura de la Revolución Mexicana." *Historias 8–9. Nuevas Reflexiones sobre la Revolución Mexicana*. Mexico City: Instituto Nacional de Antropología e Historia, 1985.

———. "On Civic Monuments and their Spectators." In *Mexican Monuments; Strange Encounters*, edited by Helen Escobedo. New York: Abbeville Press, 1989.

———. "Sobre tu capital, cada hora vuela." *Asamblea de ciudades. Años 20s-50s. Ciudad de México*. Mexico City: Museo del Palacio de Bellas Artes, 1992.

———. "La hora cívica. De monumentos cívicos y sus espectadores." *Los Rituales del Caos*. Mexico City: Ediciones Era, 1995.
Monteforte Toledo, Mario. *Las piedras vivas. Escultura y sociedad en México*. Mexico City: Instituto de Investigaciones Sociales – Universidad Nacional Autónoma de México,1979.
Montellano, Francisco. *C.B. Waite, fotógrafo. Una mirada diversa sobre el México de principios de siglo*. Mexico City; Grijalbo, 1994.
Mora, José María Luis. *Memoria que para informar sobre el origen y estado actual de las obras emprendidas para el desagüe de las lagunas del valle de México, presentó a la Excma. Diputación Provincial el Vocal Dr. D. José María Luis Mora, comisionado para reconocerlas*. Mexico City: Imprenta de la Aguila, 1823.
Morales, María Dolores. "La expansión de la ciudad de México en el siglo XIX. El caso de los fraccionamientos." In *Investigaciones sobre la historia de la ciudad de México*. Cuadernos de Trabajo del Departamento de Investigaciones Históricas. Mexico City: Instituto Nacional de Antropología e Historia, 1974.
———. "La expansión de la ciudad de México en el siglo XIX. El caso de los fraccionamientos." In *Ciudad de México. Ensayo de construcción de una historia*, edited by Alejandra Moreno Toscano. Mexico City: Instituto Nacional de Antropología e Historia – Seminario de Historia Urbana, Colección Científica 61, 1978.
———. "Francisco Somera y el primer fraccionamiento de la ciudad de México." In *Formación y desarrollo de la burguesia en México*, edited by Ciro Cardoso. Mexico City: Siglo XXI, 1978a.
———. "La expansion de la ciudad de Mexico (1858–1910)." In *Atlas de la Ciudad de México*, edited by Gustavo Garza. Mexico City: Departamento del Distrito Federal – El Colegio de México, 1987.
Moreno Toscano, Alejandra. "Cambios en los patrones de urbanización en México, 1810–1910." *Historia Mexicana* 22 (1972): 160–87.
———. "Introducción. Un ensayo de historia urbana." In *Ciudad de México: Ensayo de construcción de una historia*, edited by Alejandra Moreno Toscano. Mexico City: Instituto Nacional de Antropología e Historia – Seminario de Historia Urbana, Colección Científica 61, 1978.
———. "La constitución del espacio urbano." In *Ciudad de México. Ensayo de construcción de una historia,* edited by Alejandra Moreno Toscano. Mexico City: Instituto Nacional de Antropología e Historia – Seminario de Historia Urbana, Colección Científica 61, 1978a.
Morse, Richard M. "Cities as People." In *Rethinking the Latin American City*, edited by Jorge E. Hardoy and Richard M. Morse. Baltimore: Johns Hopkins University Press, 1992.
Mort, Frank. *Dangerous Sexualities. Medico-Moral Politics in England since 1830*. 2nd ed. London and New York: Routledge, 1987.
Murdock, Carl. "Physicians, the State and Public Health in Chile, 1881–1891." *Journal of Latin American Studies* 27 (1995): 551–67.
Murilho de Carvalho, José. *A forma âo das almas. O imaginário da República no Brasil*. São Paulo: Companhia das Letras, 1990.
Musset, Alain. *De l'eau vive à l'eau morte. Enjeux techniques et culturels dans la vallée de Mexico (XVIe-XIXe siécles)*. Paris: Editions Recherche sur les Civilisations, 1991.
Nash, Joe. *El Paseo de la Reforma: A Guide*. Mexico City: Raul Esquivel, 1959.

Needell, Jeffrey D. "The *Revolta Contra Vacina* of 1904: The Revolt Against Modernization in *Belle-Époque* Rio de Janeiro." *Hispanic American Historical Review*, no. 67 (1987): 233-69.
Nora, Pierre, ed. *Les lieux de mémoire I. La République*. Paris: Bibliothèque illustrée des histories – Gallimard, 1984.
Novo, Salvador. *Un año hace ciento. La ciudad de México en 1873*. Mexico City: Editorial Porrúa, 1973.
O'Malley, Ilene Virginia. *The Myth of the Revolution: Hero Cults and the Institutionalization of the Mexican State, 1920–1940*. New York: Greenwood Press, 1986.
Orvañanos, Domingo. *Ensayo de geografía médica y climatológica de la República Mexicana*. Mexico City: Oficina Tipográfica de la Secretaría de Fomento, 1889.
Pacheco, José Emilio. *Diario de Federico Gamboa (1892–1939)*. Prólogo, selección y notas de José Emilio Pacheco. Mexico City: Siglo XXI, 1977.
Pani, Alberto J. *La higiene en México*. Mexico City: Imprenta de J. Ballescá, 1916.
Parent-Duchâtelet, Alexandre. *La prostitution à Paris au XIXe siècle* (1836). Texte présenté et annoté para Alain Corbin. Paris: L'Univers Historique Seuil, 1981.
Payno, Manuel. *Los bandidos de Río Frío*. Mexico City: Editorial Porrúa, 1964.
Peeling, Margaret. "Contagion/germ theory/specificity." In *Companion Encyclopedia of the History of Medicine*, edited by William F. Bynum and Roy Porter. Vol. 1. London: Routledge, 1993.
Peñafiel, Antonio. *Memoria sobre las aguas potables en México*. Mexico City: Oficina Tipográfica de la Secretaría de Fomento, 1884.
———. *Explicación del edificio mexicano para la Exposición Internacional de París en 1889*. Mexico City: 1889.
Pérez Tamayo, Ruy. *El concepto de enfermedad. Su evolución a través de la historia*. 2 vols. Mexico City: Conacyt – Fondo de Cultura Económica-Universidad Nacional Autónoma de México, 1988.
Perló Cohen, Manuel, ed. *La modernización de las ciudades en México*. Mexico City: Instituto de Investigaciones Sociales – Universidad Nacional Autónoma de México, 1990.
———. *El paradigma porfiriano. Historia del desagüe del valle de México*. México: Porrúa, 1999.
Piccato, Pablo. "'El Paso de Venus por el disco del Sol'; Criminality and Alcoholism in the Late Porfiriato." *Mexican Studies/Estudios Mexicanos* 2, no. 2 (Summer 1995): 203–41.
———. *City of Suspects: Crime in Mexico City, 1900–1931*. Durham: Duke University Press, 2001.
Pineo, Ron F. "Misery and Death in the Pearl of the Pacific: Health Care in Guayaquil, Ecuador, 1870–1925." *Hispanic American Historical Review* 70, no. 4 (1990): 609–37.
Pinkney, David. *Napoleon III and the Rebuilding of Paris*. Princeton, New Jersey: Princeton University Press, 1958.
Pletcher, David M. *Rails, Mines and Progress*. Port Washington: Kennikat, 1972.
Porter, Dorothy. "Public Health." In *Companion Encyclopedia of the History of Medicine*, edited by William F. Bynum and Roy Porter. Vol. 2. London: Routledge, 1993.
Porter, Dorothy, ed. *The History of Public Health and the Modern State*. Amsterdam – Atlanta: Editions Rodopi, 1994.

Porter, Roy. "Religion and Medicine." In *Companion Encyclopedia of the History of Medicine*, edited by Roy Porter and William F. Bynum. Vol. 2. London: Routledge, 1993.

Prantl, Adolfo and José Groso. *La ciudad de México: Novísima guía universal de la capital de la república mexicana*. Mexico City: Juan Buxó y Compañía editores, Librería Madrileña, 1901.

Prashad, Vijay. "Native Dirt/Imperial Ordure: The Cholera of 1832 and the Morbid Resolutions of Modernity." *Journal of Historical Sociology* 7, no. 3 (1994): 243–60.

Prieto, Guillermo. *Memoria de mis tiempos*. Mexico City: Librería de Charles Bouret, 1906.

Programas para los trabajos del Instituto Médico Nacional en el año de 1895. Mexico City: Oficina Tipográfica de la Secretaría de Fomento, 1895.

Quevedo, Miguel Angel de. *Espacios libres y reservas forestales de las ciudades, su adaptación á jardines, parques y lugares de juego, su aplicación a la Ciudad de México*. Mexico City: Gomy Busón, 1911.

Rabasa, Emilio. *El Cuarto Poder y Moneda Falsa*. Mexico City: Editorial Porrúa, 1970.

Radkau, Verena. "Imágenes de la mujer en la sociedad porfirista. Viejos mitos en ropaje nuevo." *Revista Encuentro. El Colegio de Jalisco* 4, no. 3 (1987): 5–39.

———. "Hacia la construcción del 'eterno femenino'. El discurso científico del Porfiriato al servicio de una sociedad disciplinaria." *Papeles de la Casa Chata* 6, no. 8 (1991): 23–34.

Raigosa, Genaro. *Discurso pronunciado por el Sr. Senador Genaro Raigosa en la sesión del 16 de noviembre de 1881 sobre el contrato celebrado entre el Secretario de Fomento y el Sr. Antonio de Mier y Celis para el desagüe y saneamiento de la ciudad y del Valle de México*. Mexico City: Imprenta del Gobierno en Palacio, 1881.

Ramos Escandón, Carmen, ed. *Presencia y transparencia: La mujer en la historia de México*. Mexico City: El Colegio de México, 1992.

Ramsey, Matthew. "The Politics of Professional Monopoly in Nineteenth-Century Medicine: The French Model and Its Rivals." In *Professions and the French State, 1700–1900*, edited by Gerald L. Geison. Philadelphia: University of Pennsylvania Press, 1984.

Reese, Thomas F., and Carol McMichael Reese. "Revolutionary Urban Legacies: Porfirio Díaz's Celebrations of the Centennial of Mexican Independence in 1910." In *Estudios de Arte y Estética 37. XVII Coloquio Internacional de Historia del Arte. Arte, Historia e Identidad en América: Visiones Comparativas*. Vol. 2. Mexico City: Instituto de Investigaciones Estéticas – Universidad Nacional Autónoma de México, 1994.

Reid, Donald. *Paris Sewers and Sewermen. Realities and Representations*. Cambridge, Massachusetts: Harvard University Press, 1991.

Reseña histórica y estadística de los ferrocarriles de jurisdicción federal desde el 1 de enero de 1895 hasta el 31 de diciembre de 1899. Mexico City: Tipografía de la Dirección General de Telégrafos Federales, 1900.

Richmond, Douglas Wertz. *Venustiano Carranza's Nationalist Struggle, 1893–1920*. Lincoln: University of Nebraska Press, 1983.

Riedel, Emil. *Practical Guide of the City and Valley of Mexico*. Mexico City: I. Epstein, 1892.

Ríos Elizondo, Roberto. *Apuntes para una historia de las inundaciones de la ciudad de México*. Mexico City: Boletín de la Sociedad Mexicana de Geografía y Estadística, 1954.

Rivera Cambas, Manuel. *México pintoresco, artístico y monumental*. Mexico City: Imprenta de la Reforma, 1883.

Rodríguez, Martha Eugenia. "Semanarios, gacetas, revistas y periódicos médicos del siglo XIX mexicano." *Boletín del Instituto de Investigaciones Bibliográficas – Nueva época* 2, no. 2 (1997): 61–96.

_____. *Contaminación e insalubridad en la ciudad de México en el siglo XVIII*. Mexico City: Departamento de Historia y Filosofía de la Medicina – Universidad Nacional Autónoma de México, 2000.

Rodríguez O. Jaime E. *El proceso de la Independencia de México*. Mexico City: Instituto de Investigaciones Dr. José María Luis Mora, 1992.

Rodríguez de Romo, Ana Cecilia. "La ciencia pasteuriana a través de la vacuna antirrábica: el caso mexicano." *DYNAMIS* 16 (1996): 291–316.

Rodríguez Prampolini, Ida. "La figura del indio en la pintura del siglo XIX: fondo ideológico." In *La polémica del arte nacional en México, 1850–1910*, edited by Daniel Schávelzon. Mexico City: Fondo de Cultura Económica, 1988.

Rogers, Naoemi. "Germs with Legs: Flies, Disease and the New Public Health." *Bulletin of the History of Medicine* 63 (1989): 599–617.

Romero, José Luis. *Latinoamerica: Las ciudades y las ideas*. Mexico City: Siglo XXI, 1976.

Romero Flores, Jesús. *México: Historia de una gran ciudad*. Mexico City: Editorial Botas, 1953.

Rosen, George. *A History of Public Health*. Expanded edition, introduction by Elizabeth Fee. Baltimore and London: Johns Hopkins University Press, 1993.

Rosenberg, Charles. *The Cholera Years: The United States in 1832, 1849 and 1866. With a new Afterword*. Chicago and London: University of Chicago Press, 1987.

Ruiz, Luis E. *Tratado elemental de pedagogía*. Mexico City: Oficina Tipográfica de la Secretaría de Fomento, 1900.

_____. *Cartilla de higiene; profilaxis de las enfermedades transmisibles para la enseñanza primaria*. Paris: Vda. de Ch. Bouret, 1903.

_____. *Tratado elemental de higiene*. Mexico City: Oficina Tipográfica de la Secretaría de Fomento, 1904.

_____. *Guia de la ciudad de México*. Mexico City: Imprenta del Gobierno Federal, 1910.

SAHOP. *500 Planos de la ciudad de México, 1325–1933*. Mexico City: Secretaría de Asentamientos Urbanos y Obras Públicas, 1982.

Salazar, José Guillermo. "Supersticiones y creencias vulgares en los países de Hispano-América." In *Memoria de la Sociedad Científica 'Antonio Alzate'. Revista Científica y Bibliográfica* 32, nos. 5–9 (1911–12): 427–33.

Saldaña, Juan José and Luz Fernanda Azuela. "De amateurs a profesionales. Las sociedades científicas mexicanas en el siglo XIX." *Quipu. Revista Latinoamericana de Historia de las Ciencias y la Tecnología* 11, no. 2 (May–August 1994): 135–72.

Salessi, Jorge. *Médicos maleantes y maricas. Higiene, criminología y homosexualidad en la construcción de la nación Argentina. (Buenos Aires: 1871–1914)*. Buenos Aires: Estudios Culturales – Beatriz Viterbo Editora, 1995.

Sánchez, Jesús. "Higiene de los jardines públicos y particulares de la ciudad de México." *Gaceta Médica de México* 21, no. 3 (1 February 1886): 45–53, 74–78.

Sariol, Florentino. *Ligeras consideraciones acerca de la influencia nociva que ejercen las materias fecales sobre la salubridad: medidas higiénicas para combatir dicha influencia.* Mexico City: Imprenta de Francisco Díaz de León, 1887.

Schávelzon, Daniel. "El primer monumento a Cuauhtémoc (1869)." In *La polémica del arte nacional en México, 1850–1910*, edited by Daniel Schávelzon. Mexico City: Fondo de Cultura Económica, 1988.

———. "Notas sobre Manuel Vilar y sus esculturas de Moctezuma y Tlahuicole." In *La polémica del arte nacional en México, 1850–1910*, edited by Daniel Schávelzon. Mexico City: Fondo de Cultura Económica, 1988a.

Schendel, Gordon. *Medicine in Mexico. From Aztec Herbs to Betatrons.* Austin: University of Texas Press, 1968.

Schorske, Carl E. *Fin-de-siècle Vienna: Politics and Culture.* New York: Vintage Books, 1981.

Schultz, Stanley K., and Clay McShane. "To Engineer the Metropolis: Sewers, Sanitation, and City Planning in Late-Nineteenth-Century America." *Journal of American History* 65, no. 2 (September 1978): 389–411.

———. "Pollution and Political Reform in Urban America: The Role of Municipal Engineers, 1840–1920." In *Pollution and Reform in American Cities, 1870–1930*, edited by Martin V. Melosi. Austin and London: University of Texas Press, 1980.

Scobie, James. *Buenos Aires: Plaza to Suburb, 1870–1910.* New York: Oxford University Press, 1974.

Sedano, Francisco. *Noticias de México recogidas desde el año de 1756. Coordinadas, escritas de nuevo y puestas por orden alfabético en 1800. Prólogo de Joaquín García Icazbalceta.* Mexico City: n.p, 1880.

Sevcenko, Nicolau. *A Revolta da Vacina. Mentes insanas em corpos rebeldes.* São Paulo: Editora Scipione, 1993.

Sierra, Carlos. *Breve historia de la navegación en la ciudad de México.* Mexico City: Departamento del Distrito Federal, 1984.

Sierra, Justo. *Evolución política del pueblo Mexicano.* Obras Completas del Maestro Justo Sierra. Vol. 13. Mexico City: Universidad Nacional Autónoma de México, 1957.

Silva, Máximo. *Higiene popular. Colección de conocimientos y consejos indispensables para evitar las enfermedades y prolongar la vida, arreglada para uso de las familias.* Mexico City: Departamento de Talleres Gráficos, 1917.

Soja, Edward. *Postmodern Geographies: The Reassertion of Space in Critical Social Theory.* London: Verso, 1989.

Soja, Edward and B. Hooper. "The Spaces that Difference Makes: Some Notes on the Geographical Margins of the New Cultural Policies." In *Place and Politics of Identity*, edited by Michael Keith and Steve Pile. London: Routledge, 1993.

Sosa, Francisco. *Apuntamientos para la historia del monumento a Cuauhtémoc.* Mexico City: Oficina Tipográfica de la Secretaría de Fomento, 1887.

———. *Las estatuas de la Reforma: notas biográficas de los personajes en ellas representados.* Mexico City: Oficina Tipográfica de la Secretaría de Fomento, 1900.

Speckman Guerra, Elisa. *Crimen y castigo. Legislación penal, interpretaciones de la criminalidad y administración de justicia (Ciudad de México, 1871–1910).* Mexico City: El Colegio de México – Universidad Nacional Autónoma de México, 2002.

Staples, Anne. "*Policia y Buen Gobierno*: Municipal Efforts to Regulate Public Behaviour, 1821–1857." In *Rituals of Rule, Rituals of Resistance. Public Celebrations and Popular Culture in Mexico*, edited by William Beezley, Cheryl English Martin and William E. French. Wilmington: Scholarly Resources, 1994.

Stepan, Nancy Leys. *The Hour of Eugenics. Race, Gender and Nation in Latin America*. Ithaca, N.Y.: Cornell University Press, 1991.

Stevens, Donald F. "Temerse la ira del cielo: los conservadores y la religiosidad popular en los tiempos del cólera." In *El conservadurismo mexicano en el siglo XIX (1810–1910)*, coordinated by Humberto Morales and William Fowler. Mexico: Benemérita Universidad Autónoma de Puebla – University of Saint Andrews, 1999.

Szuchman, Mark D. "The City as Vision – The Development of Urban Culture in Latin America." In *I Saw a City Invincible. Urban Portraits on Latin America*, edited by Joseph M. Gilbert and Mark Szuchman. Delaware: Jaguar Books on Latin America – Scholarly Resources, 1996.

Tate Lanning, John. *The Royal Protomedicato. The Regulation of the Medical Professions in the Spanish Empire*, edited by John Jay Te Paske. Durham: Duke University Press, 1985.

Tellez Pizarro, Manuel. *Estudios sobre cimientos para los edificios de la ciudad de México*. Mexico City: Tipografía de la Dirección de Telégrafos Federales, 1907.

Tello Peón, Berta. "Intención decorativa en los objetos de uso cotidiano de los interiores domésticos del porfiriato." In *El arte y la vida cotidiana. XVI Coloquio Internacional de Historia del Arte*. Mexico City: Instituto de Investigaciones Estéticas, Universidad Nacional Autónoma de México, 1995.

Temkin, Owsei. *The Double Face of Janus and Other Essays in the History of Medicine*. London: Johns Hopkins University Press, 1977.

Tenenbaum, Barbara. "Murals in Stone. The Paseo de la Reforma and Porfirian Mexico, 1873–1910." In *La ciudad y el campo en la historia de México. Papers presented at the VII Conference of Mexican and the Unites States Historians, Oaxaca, 1985*. Vol. 1. Mexico City: Universidad Nacional Autónoma de México, 1992.

——. "Streetwise History: The Paseo de la Reforma and the Porfirian State, 1876–1910." In *Rituals of Rule, Rituals of Resistance. Public Celebrations and Popular Culture in Mexico*, edited by William Beezley, Cheryl English Martin and William E. French. Wilmington: Scholarly Resources, 1994.

Tenorio Trillo, Mauricio. "1910 Mexico City: Space and Nation in the City of the Centenario." *Journal of Latin American Studies* 28, part 1 (February 1996): 75–104.

Tenorio Trillo, Mauricio. *Mexico at the World's Fairs. Crafting a Modern Nation*. Berkeley: University of California Press, 1996.

Terres, José. "Influencia del desagüe del Valle de México en la higiene de la capital." In *Estudios referentes a la desecación del lago de Texcoco, año de 1895*. Mexico City: Oficina Tipográfica de la Secretaría de Fomento, 1895.

The Concise Oxford Dictionary of Art and Artists, edited by I. Chilvers. Oxford: Oxford University Press, 1992.

Tomes, Nancy. "The Private Side of Public Health: Sanitary Scienc, Domestic Hygiene, and the Germ Theory, 1870–1900." *Bulletin of the History of Medicine* 64 (1990): 509–39.

———. *The Gospel of Germs. Men, Women, and the Microbe in American Life*. Cambridge, Massachusetts: Harvard University Press, 1998.

Topik, Steven. "The Economic Role of the State in Liberal Regimes: Brazil and Mexico Compared, 1880–1910." In *Guiding the Invisible Hand. Economic Liberalism and the State in Latin American History*, edited by Joseph Love and Nils Jacobsen. New York: Praeger, 1988.

———. "Economic Domination by the Capital: Mexico City and Rio de Janeiro, 1888–1910." In *La ciudad y el campo en la historia de México. Papers presented at the VII Conference of Mexican and the United States Historians*. Oaxaca, 1985. Vol. 1. Mexico City: Universidad Nacional Autónoma de México, 1992.

Tornel, Manuel. *Guía práctica del viajero y del comerciante en México*. Mexico City: Librería de la Enseñanza, 1987.

Tovar de Teresa, Guillermo. *La Ciudad de los Palacios: Crónica de un patrimonio perdido*. Vol. 1. Mexico City: Editorial Vuelta, 1992.

Tuñón Pablos, Enriqueta et al. *El álbum de la mujer. Antología ilustrada de las mexicanas. El Porfiriato y la Revolución*. Vol. 4. Mexico City: Instituto Nacional de Antropología e Historia, 1991.

Unikel, Luis. *La dinámica del crecimiento de la ciudad de México*. Mexico City: Fundación para Estudios de la Población, A.C., 1972.

Urías Horcasitas, Beatríz. *Indígena y criminal. Interpretaciones del derecho y la antropología en México, 1871–1921*. Mexico City: Universidad Iberoamericana, 2000.

Urquiaga, Juan. "La arquitectura en México. Porfiriato y movimiento moderno." *México en el Arte. Nueva Epoca* 1 (1983): 41–48.

Valadés, José. *El Porfirismo. El crecimiento*. Mexico City: Universidad Nacional Autónoma de México. 2 vols. 1977.

———. *El Porfirismo. Historia de un régimen. El Nacimiento*. Vol. 1. Mexico City: Universidad Nacional Autónoma de México, 1987.

Vallejo, Hilarión. *La penitenciaría en México desde el punto de vista de la higiene*. Mexico City: Guadalupana, 1907.

Vargas Salguero, Ramón. "Las fiestas del Centenario: recapitulaciones y vaticinios." In *La arquitectura mexicana del siglo XX*, edited by Fernando González Gortazar. Mexico City: Consejo Nacional para la Cultura y las Artes, 1994.

Velasco, Pilar. "La epidemia de cólera de 1833 y la mortalidad en la ciudad de México." *Estudios Demográficos y Urbanos* 19 (1992): 95–135.

Velázquez-Guadarrama, Angélica. "La historia patria en el Paseo de la Reforma. La propuesta de Francisco Sosa y la consolidación del estado en el Porfiriato." In *Estudios de Arte y Estética 37. XVII Coloquio Internacional de Historia del Arte. Arte, Historia e Identidad en América: Visiones Comparativas*. Mexico City: Instituto de Investigaciones Estéticas – Universidad Nacional Autónoma de México, 1994.

Viera, Juan de. "Breve compendiosa narración de la ciudad de México, corte y cabeza de toda la América septentrional (1777)." In *La ciudad de México en el siglo XVIII (1690–1780). Tres crónicas*, edited by Antonio Rubial García. Mexico City: Consejo Nacional para la Cultura y las Artes, 1990.

Vigarello, Georges. *Le propre et le sale. L'hygiène du corps depuis le Moyen Age*. Paris: Editions Seuil, 1985.

Violich, Francis. "Mexico City and Mexico. Two Cultural Worlds in Perspective." *Third World Planning Review* 3, no. 4 (1983): 361–86.

Villarroel, Hipólito. *Enfermedades políticas que padece la capital de esta Nueva España en casi todos los cuerpos de que se compone y remedios que se le deben aplicar para su curación si se quiere que sea útil al rey y al público* (first published in 1785). Mexico City: Colección Tlahuicole 2, Editorial Porrúa, 1982.

Viqueira Albán, Juan Pedro. *¿Relajados o reprimidos? Diversiones públicas y vida social en la ciudad de México durante el Siglo de las Luces.* Mexico City: Fondo de Cultura Económica, 1995.

Voekel, Pamela. "Peeing on the Palace: Bodily Resistance to Bourbon Reforms in Mexico City." *Journal of Historical Sociology* 5, no. 2 (1992): 183–208.

———. "Piety and Public Space: The Cemetery Campaign in Veracruz, 1789–1810." In *Latin American Popular Culture. An Introduction*, edited by William H. Beezley and Linda A. Curcio-Nagy. Wilmington, Delaware: Scholarly Resources, 2000.

Warner, Marina. *Monuments and Maidens: The Allegory of the Female Form.* London: Picador, 1985.

Weeks, Charles. *The Juárez Myth in Mexico.* Alabama: University of Alabama Press, 1987.

Williams, Marilyn T. *"The Great Unwashed": Public Baths in Urban America, 1840–1920.* Columbus: Ohio State University Press, 1991.

Wilsford, Daniel. *Doctors and the State: The Politics of Health Care in France and the United States.* Durham: Duke University Press, 1991.

Woods, Robert and John Woodward, eds. *Urban Disease and Mortality in Nineteenth-Century England.* New York: St. Martin's Press, 1984.

Index

Academia de Bellas Artes, 98
Academia de San Carlos, 98
Academia Nacional de Medicina
    (National Academy of Medicine),
    39, 131, 132
Agea, Ramón, 98
Ahuítzotl (Aztec king)
    criticisms of, 101–2
    as landmark or signal, 91
    neo pre-hispanic style and, 84, 98, 108
    statue on Paseo de la Viga, 101
    statue on Paseo de la Reforma, 91,
        100
    See also Indios Verdes, Itzcóatl
Alamán, Lucas, 120
Alameda, 11, 79, 104
Alciati, Enrique, 106, 108
alcoholism
    and criminality, 68
    during late-colonial period, 13
    during late nineteenth century, 68
    as a social disease, 136
Alfaro, Jesús, 40
Almada, Vicente, 111
Alzate, José Antonio de, 8
Amazonas (street), 83
American Dredging Company, 128

Americana (*colonia*), 46, 83
Ampliación San Rafael – La Blanca
    (*colonia*), 46
Ampliación Santa María – Ladrillera
    (*colonia*), 46
aqueducts
    Arcos de Belem, 102–3
    Chapultepec, 103
    drainage system and, 129
    lack of maintenance, 15, 17–19, 54
    threats to health and, 6, 17, 35, 41,
        54, 102–3
    urban reforms and, 17–19, 102, 114
Arcos de Belem, 102–3
Argentina, 61, 74
Armed Forces College (Colegio
    Militar), 24
Armed Forces Medical School (Escuela
    Práctico-Médico Militar), 24
Arquitectos (*colonia*), 46, 48, 49
Asociación Metodófila Gabino Barreda,
    39
Atlampa (pueblo), 74
Austria, 80
Avenida de Hombres Ilustres (street), 144
Avenida de Pachuca (river), 32
Aznar, Marcial, 104

*B*acteriology, 37, 145, 146, 149, 169n48, 169n52, 192n116. *See also* disease causation
Bagally, Santiago, 97
Balbuena Park, 41
Baltimore, 116
Baratillo (market), 66
Barreda, Gabino, 165n4
Barroso (*colonia*), 46, 48
bathing
   at-home, 41, 42, 69, 70
   bathing establishments, 41, 69
   germ theory of disease and, 42, 147
   urban poor and, 69, 70, 148
   See also water
Battle of Puebla, 79
Bello Pérez, Eduardo, 142
Beltrán y Puga, Guillermo, 107, 111
Berlin, 131, 144
Berlín (street), 83
Bernáldez, Francisco de P., 70, 71
Boari, Adamo, 84
Body, John, 128
Boletín del Consejo Superior de Salubridad del Distrito Federal (magazine), 60
Branciforte, Miguel de la Grúa Talamanca y, 15
Braniff family, 84
Bravo, Nicolás, 107, 108
Brehme, Hugo, 82
Britain, 20, 29, 51, 128
Brussels, 131
Budapest, 144
Buenos Aires, 51, 54
Bustamante, Carlos María de, 162n47
Bustamante, Anastasio, 20

*C*alderón, Francisco, 118
Calzada Degollado (street), 80
Cámara de Senadores (Chamber of Senators), 31
Campeche, 142
canals
   Canal de La Viga, 82, 127, 134
   Canal de San Lázaro, 34–35, 82, 130
   drainage of, 48
   inspection of, 59
   threats to health and, 10, 11, 54
Carlota (empress of Mexico), 79

Carranza, Venustiano, 148–50
Casarín, Alejandro, 98, 100
Castera, Ignacio, 17, 18
census, 16, 28, 61
Centennial Celebrations of Mexico's Independence, 96, 112
   cleanliness during, 110–13, 145
   public health during, 143
   monument to Juárez and, 105
   monument to Independence and, 109–10
   Popular Hygiene Exhibition and, 67, 113, 144, 145
Centro Mercantil (store), 82
Cerralvo, Pacheco de Osorio Rodrigo – Viceroy and Marquis, 118
Cervantes de Salazar, Francisco, 7
Chamber of Deputies (Cámara de Diputados), 86, 87
Chamber of Senators (Cámara de Senadores), 31
Chapultepec
   aqueduct, 103
   forest of, 52, 86, 87, 103
   castle of, 79
Charles III (Spain), 2, 9
Charles IV (Spain), 16
   statue of, 80, 108
Chavero, Alfredo, 99
Chicago International Exhibition, 95
Chimalistac (pueblo), 136
Chile, 61
Chopo (*colonia*), 46
Churubusco (pueblo), 111
Cinco de Mayo (street), 52
Cintura (railroad station), 49
Coahuila, 26
Código Sanitario de los Estados Unidos Mexicanos. *See* sanitary code
Colegio Militar (Armed Forces College), 24
Colón, Cristóbal (statue), 81, 95, 108
colonial (Bourbon period), xv–xvi, 1–22
   cleanliness during, 2, 4, 9, 17
   enlightenment reforms, xvi, 2–3, 6, 9
   epidemics, 4–5
   images of ideal city, 2, 6, 7–8, 14, 17–18, 28
   good government or *policía*, 2, 8, 11, 13, 14, 17

Index

medical discourse during, 11–12
Municipal Council, 5
practice of medicine during, 5
public good, xvi, 16, 17
public health during, xvi, 4, 5, 15, 16, 17, 18, 19
public markets, 11, 14–16, 18
Royal Treasury of Mexico City, 118
sewers, 9, 10, 18
streets, 6, 8–11, 14–18
urban pathologies, 6–7, 13–14
urban projects, 2–3, 8, 4–11, 15–17
urban sanitation, 14–18
See also drainage, floods, Revillagigedo
colonias, 45–52, 74, 76, 82, 83, 94, 133, 157
and urban expansion, 45–52
and lower-class, 52–53
See also names of individual *colonias*
Commission of Public Works (Dirección General de Obras Públicas), 124
Condesa (*colonia*), 46, 51, 83
Condesa (hacienda), 83
Condorcet, Antoine Caritat, marquis of, 2
Contreras, Jesús F., 98
Contreras, Manuel María, 125, 130
Cooper, Donald, 4, 5
Corbin, Alain, 4, 36, 133
Cordero, Juan, 98
Cordier, Charles Henri Joseph, 95
Correos (building), 84, 86, 87
Cortés, Hernán, 152
Cosmes, Francisco G., 25
Council of Indies (Spain), 18
Cowdray, Lord. *See* Pearson, Sir Weetman
Coyoacán (pueblo), 111
crime
control of the environment and, 33–34
alcoholism and, 68
as social disease, 152, 171n5
Croix, Carlos Francisco de, marquis viceroy, 14
Cuartelito (*colonia*), 46
Cuauhtémoc (*colonia*), 56, 51, 52, 83
Cuauhtémoc (emperor of the Aztecs) 90, 94, 99, 106

Cuauhtémoc's monument, 94, 99–100
1877 decree and, 97–101
monumental space and, 110–11
neo pre-hispanic style and, 84, 97, 108
Cuauhtemotzin (street), 111
Cuautitlán (river), 32, 117, 119

David, Jacques-Louis, 98
Delacroix, Jacques Vincent, 7
Desagüe. *See* drainage system
Díaz, Porfirio
government of, xii, xvii, 58
and order and progress, 23, 25, 87, 92
and monument to Cuauhtémoc, 99–100
and monument to Benito Juárez, 104–6
and drainage system, 126, 138–39
and sewage system, 134
See also Mexico City, monuments, Porfiriato, public health
Díaz de León (*colonia*), 46, 49
Díaz Lombardo, Isidro, 122
Díaz Mirón, Salvador, 109
Dinamarca (street), 83
Dirección General de Instrucción Primaria (General Board of Primary Education), 39
Dirección General de Obras Públicas (Commission of Public Works), 111, 112, 124
disease causation, xiv, 3–4
air pollution, xiv; 4, 6, 35, 70, 132
atmospheric-miasmatic theory, xiv, 3, 6, 10, 11, 15–17, 22, 23, 30, 34, 36–38, 132–33, 145, 158
bad odours and, 4, 22, 23, 34, 35, 55, 56, 68, 75, 133, 138, 145, 148, 157
germ theory of, 21, 36, 37, 42, 65, 66, 131, 132, 141, 146, 148, 149, 156, 169n52, 170n74, 170n75
lack of morality and, 22, 23, 34, 71
overcrowding and, 6, 30, 37, 66, 68–71, 75, 132, 145, 148, 150
prostitution and, 136–38
urban pathologies, 6–7, 11–13
urban poor and, 30, 70–73, 132, 150–51, 155
See also bacteriology

diseases
  bronchitis, 66
  cervical cancer, 136
  cholera, 19, 20, 29, 37, 65–66, 69, 70, 125; epidemic of 1833, 19–20, 164n84, 87, 88
  smallpox, 4, 5, 37, 39, 64–66, 69, 72
  social, 151–52
  tuberculosis, 66, 69, 142, 145
  typhoid, 37, 66, 69, 146
  typhus, 4, 5, 62, 65, 66, 69, 72, 73, 131
  zymotic, 37
disinfection, 40, 62, 69, 144
  use of disinfectants, 123, 132
Dondé Preciat, Emilio, 97
Douglas, Mary, 42
drainage, drainage system
  colonial period, 14, 117–19
  construction of, 125–26, 127–29
  control of the environment and, xiii-xiv, xvi, 115, 116, 139
  drainage of Huehuetoca, 14, 117–19, 139
  foreign investment, 125
  Gran Canal de Desagüe, 120–22, 124, 127–29, 133, 140, 144
  idea of progress and, 120, 123, 139
  image of modern city and, xv, 57, 115, 122, 139–40
  inauguration of, 138–39, 140, 144
  Junta Directiva del Desagüe del Valle de México, 126, 127
  monument to, 140, 181n49
  neglect of, 120
  objectives of, 127, 128
  physical expansion of the city and, 40, 128
  1856 project, 120–22
  as a public health work, 125
  public visits to, 141
  resources invested in, 85–86, 86 (table 4), 119, 128
  sewage system and, 130–33
  See also floods, sewers

*E*l Imparcial (newspaper), 100, 135, 138, 141, 148
El Imparcial (*colonia*) 46

El Mundo (newspaper), 68
El Mundo Científico (magazine), 27
El Municipio Libre (newspaper), 70, 76, 125
El Siglo XIX (newspaper), 98
El Tiempo (newspaper), 126
El Universal (newspaper), 77
England, 29, 38, 61
Escandón, Antonio, 81, 93, 95
Escuela Nacional de Medicina (National School of Medicine), 24, 40
Escuela Práctico-Médica Militar (Armed Forces Medical School), 24
Escuela de Salubridad Pública, 153
Esparza, Rosendo, 122, 126, 127
Espinosa, Luis, 122, 123, 125, 127, 130, 131
Europe, 29, 60, 91, 104
Exposition Universelle de Paris (1889), 89, 100

*F*ernández, Justino, 95
Fernández, Leandro, 130
First National Congress of Physicians (1876), 65
Flandrau, Charles, 113
floods, 31
  colonial period and, 18, 117–19
  criticisms and complaints, 126–27
  in Holland, 124
  during pre-Hispanic period, 117
  during the nineteenth century, 54–55, 119, 120, 126
  threat of, 14, 15, 21, 31, 32, 33, 34, 35, 50, 115–16, 157
  See also drainage, sewers, water
Florence, 108
Flores, Leopoldo, 112
Fonssagrives (French physician), 39
food and drink
  adulteration of, 69
  commercialization of, 9, 68
  inspection of, 59
  Sanitary Code (1891) and, 61
fountains
  "5th of May" fountain, 79
  public fountains, 35, 41, 123

France
  medical gaze in, 6
  paving system, 14
  prostitution in, 136
  recycling of urban waste in, 133
  sanitary engineering in, 116
Franco, Alonso, 118
Franz Josef (emperor of Austria), 80
French Empire (in Mexico, 1864–67), 79
French Revolution, 98
Fuente, Manuel de la, 37

Galen, 3, 12
Galindo y Villa, Jesús, 107
Gamboa, Federico, 136–38
Garay, Francisco de, 120, 125
García, Genaro, 143
García, Telésforo, 165n4
Gargollo y Parra, Manuel, 97
Garitas, Gonzalo, 107
Gaviño, Ángel, 141
Gayol, Roberto, 130, 131, 145
General Board of Primary Education, 39
General Hospital (Hospital General), 86, 87, 144
Germ theory, xiv, 21, 37, 42, 65, 66, 131, 132, 146, 148, 149, 158. *See also* bacteriology, disease causation
Gómez Farías, Valentín, 19
González, Ruy, 184n6
González, Manuel, xii, 125
González Obregón, Luis, 119, 122
Gortari, Hira de, 61
green areas, 11
  hygiene and, 40, 47, 150
  urban planning and, 51, 80
  urban working class and, 40–41
Groso, José, 82
Guadalupe (railroad station), 49
Guanajuato, 26
Gudiel, Francisco, 164n6
Guerra, Gabriel, 98
Guerrero (*colonia*), 46, 48–50, 73
Guerrero, Julio, 33, 68
Guerrero, Vicente, 107
Güijosa, José, 31
Gutiérrez, Rodrigo, 98
Gutiérrez Nájera, Manuel, 96

Hale, Charles, 25
Hall, Charles S., 84
Hamburgo (street), 83
Haussmann, George Eugène, 51, 80
Heredia, Guillermo de, 104
Hernández Franyutti, Regina, 61
Hidalga, Luis de la, 106
Hidalgo (*colonia*), 46, 49
Hidalgo (railroad station), 49
Hidalgo y Costilla, Miguel, 79
  monument to independence and, 94, 107, 108. *See also* monuments
Hippocrates, 3
Hoberman, Louisa, 119
Holland, 124
Hospital Juárez, 39
Huehuetoca (pueblo), 117
Humboldt, Alexander Von, 120
hygiene
  Congreso Higiénico Pedagógico (1882), 123
  Congreso Nacional de Higiene (1883), 123
  definition of, 39
  image of modern city and, 77
  moral dimension of, 43, 56, 71–72, 75–76
  private (personal), 20, 22, 23, 37, 42, 56, 60, 73, 75–76
  Popular Hygiene Exhibition, 143–47
  progress in, 116
  "religion of", 20
  social and political character of, 63–64
  urban, 39–40, 56
  urban population and, xiii, 68, 70, 71–73, 74, 132
  water and, 41
hygienic education, 23, 57, 71–72, 76, 143–45
hygienists
  areas of concern, 23–24, 25, 38–42, 43
  as advisors, xiv, 22, 27, 29, 37, 47, 146, 149
  community of, xiv, 22–25, 43, 56, 57, 71, 74, 124, 145, 146
  urban, 22, 27, 38, 39, 47, 56, 71, 74, 146

*I*ndianilla (*colonia*), 46, 49
Indios Verdes (statues), 84, 91, 98, 100–4.
  See also Ahuítzotl, Itzcóatl
Instituto Antirrábico, 69. *See also*
  vaccination
International Conferences on Hygiene,
  144
Interoceánico (railroad station), 49, 84
Islas, Manuel, 97
Italy, 139
Iturbide, Agustín de, 79
Itzcóatl (Aztec king), 84, 101, 102. *See
  also* Indios Verdes, Ahuítzotl
Izaguirre, Leandro, 98
Iztaccíhuatl (volcano), 88

*J*alisco, 26
Jiménez, Francisco, 96–98
Juárez (*colonia*), 46, 51, 52, 83, 103
Juárez, Benito
  Laws of Reform and, 78
  legacy of, 92, 182n72, 77.
  Paseo de la Reforma and, 80
  monument to, 91, 94, 104–6
  1869 monument to Cuauhtémoc
    and, 97. *See also* monuments
Junta Directiva de Beneficencia, 58, 59
Junta Directiva de las Obras del
  Desagüe, 122, 126–29, 138–40
Junta de las Obras de Saneamiento de la
  Ciudad de México, 130

*K*ahlo, Guillermo, 82
Katzman, Israel, 83
Knight, Alan, 72
Koch, Robert, 14, 37

*L*a Berge, Ann, 30
La Bolsa (*colonia*), 46, 49, 52
La Castañeda (mental asylum), 144
La Esmeralda (store), 84
La Exposición Internacional Mexicana,
  (magazine), 96
La Libertad (newspaper), 39
La Victoria (textile factory), 127
La Viga (*colonia*), 46
Ladrón de Guevara, Baltasar, 2, 7–11, 14,
  157

lake system, 32, 118–19
Lake Chalco, 32, 82
Lake Chapala, 87
Lake Mexico, 10, 32, 117
Lake San Cristóbal, 117, 120
Lake Texcoco:
  final destination of city's sewage, 22,
    31, 130, 133, 156
  inspection of, 34–35
  invasion of, 10, 35, 114, 117
  source of disease, 31, 34, 35–36, 56, 65
  threat to good order and policy, 17
  urban expansion and, 48, 50, 53–54
Lake Xochimilco, 32, 82
Lake Xaltocan, 120, 121
Lake Zumpango, 117, 120, 121
Lara y Pardo, Luis, 136
Laws of Reform (Leyes de Reforma),
  48, 78, 90, 104
León de la Barra, Francisco, 147
Le Roy Ladurie, Emmanuel, 6
Lerdo de Tejada, Sebastián, 78, 80
Liceaga, Eduardo, 28, 41, 62, 65, 144–47
Lima, 160n17
Limantour (*colonia*), 46, 49
Limantour, José Yves, 84, 126, 127
Lira, Andrés, 48
London, 9, 69, 76, 124, 125, 144
London International Exhibition
  (1851), 89
Londres (street), 83
López de Santa Anna, Antonio, 106
Lucerna (street), 83

*M*acedo, Miguel, 26, 43, 109, 126
Macedo, Pablo, 134
Madero, Francisco, 150
Madrid, 2, 9, 11
Magdalena (river), 32
Mancera, Gabriel, 126
Manso y Zúñiga, Francisco, archbishop
  of Mexico, 118
Marroquín y Rivera, Manuel, 107, 146
Martínez, Enrico, 118
Mayorga, Martín de (viceroy), 8
Maximilian (Emperor of Mexico), 79,
  80, 106
Maza (*colonia*), 49, 112
Maza, Francisco de la, 18

Index

medical education, 5, 20, 21, 24
medical journals, 21, 166n12. *See also* scientific journals
medical profession, 57, 58, 145, 153. *See also* scientific associations
medical societies, 21, 57, 16591
Medical Faculty of the Federal District (Facultad Médica del Distrito Federal), 20, 57
Medical Science Establishment (Establecimiento de Ciencias Médicas), 20, 21
Méndez, Eleuterio, 95
Méndez, Simón, 119
Mendívil, José, 19
Mercier, Louis Sébastien, 7, 161n28
Mérida, 87, 142, 143
Mexican Constitution of 1857, 61, 94, 105
Mexican Constitution of 1917, 152, 158
Mexican Revolution of 1910, xii, 147, 149, 152, 153, 192n138
Mexico City, xii, xvi, 52, 87, 124, 156–57
   architectural styles in, xvi, 78, 81, 83–84, 106
   changes during Porfiriato, 45–52, 59, 60, 64, 73, 78, 80, 83, 88, 103, 124, 128, 156
   demographic growth, 26, 45; according to 1890 census, 61 (table 2)
   environmental threats of, 31- 38
   modernization of, xv, 26, 47, 85–87, 155
   as the most unsanitary city in the world, xii, xiii, 6–7, 13–14, 130, 132, 147, 150
   as organism, 6–7, 11, 135–36
   resources allocated to, 85, 86 (table 4), 86, 87 (table 5)
   rural-urban migration, 26, 38, 47
   social boundaries in, xvi, 46, 48–53, 56, 80
   wards (cuarteles), 8, 58, 110
Mexico, Department of, 21, 57
Mexico-Tenochtitlán, 32, 88, 94, 97, 122
Michoacán, 26
Milán (street), 83
Mille, Antoine, 116, 133
Ministry of Economic Development (Mexico), 24, 79, 120, 123, 126

Ministry of the Interior (Mexico), 27, 57, 58, 59, 109, 115, 145, 147, 148, 152
Mitla, 97
Moctezuma II (statue), 98
Molina, Olegario, 142, 143
Monnet, Jerôme, 7
Monsiváis, Carlos, 88, 99
Montes de Oca, Vicente, 70
Monumento a la Revolución (Palacio Legislativo), 83
monuments, xii, xv; xvii, 1, 48, 57, 76, 77–78, 79, 81, 90–91, 94–96, 100, 101
   Cristóbal Colón, 81, 95
   Cuauhtémoc on Paseo de la Viga, 97
   as educational vehicles, 91
   and 1877 decree, 93–95
   Indios Verdes, 98, 100–1
   monument to Benito Juárez, 91, 104–6
   monument to Cuauhtémoc, 91, 98, 100, 102, 110
   monument to Independence, 79, 86, 87, 91, 94, 106–10, 112
   and pre-Hispanic past, 84, 89, 90, 97, 98, 99, 108, 113, 141
   See also Ahuítzotl, Itzcóatl, Mexico City, Paseo de la Reforma
Mora, José María Luis, 120
Morales, María Dolores, 45, 46
Morales Pereira, Samuel, 141
Morelos (*colonia*), 46, 49, 147
Morelos y Pavón, José María, 79
municipal council
   complaints against Revillagigedo, 18
   drainage system and, 125, 126
   expansion of the city and, 45–46, 51
   hygienists and, 24
   inauguration of Cuauhtémoc's monument and, 97
   lack of resources of, 49–50, 103
   public health and, 5, 21, 70, 110, 125
   of Puebla, 142
   sewage system and, 130
   statue of Revillagigedo and, 1
   Superior Sanitation Council and, 57, 58
   urban population's claims and demands towards, 103, 126–27, 134–35

*N*apoleon III, 80
National Academy of Medicine, 39, 131, 132
National Palace, 94
National School of Medicine, 24, 40
New Spain, 8, 9, 11, 12, 14, 15, 16, 17, 19, 117, 120, 157
New York, 124, 131
Nochostingo (mountains), 117
Noreña, Miguel, 98
Nueva del Paseo (*colonia*), 83

*O*bregón, José, 98
Oficina de Educación Higiénica (1922), 153
Olmos, Tiburcio, 127
Orozco, Ricardo, 124, 125
Orvañanos, Domingo, 41, 65, 70, 145

*P*alacio de Bellas Artes (Teatro Nacional), 84, 86, 87
Palacio de Hierro (store), 83
Palacio Legislativo (Chamber of Deputies), 83, 86, 87
Palenque, 97
Pan-American Congress (1901), 122
Panes, Mariano, 127
Pani, Alberto J., 149–52
Pánuco (river), 120
Parent-Duchâtelet, Alexandre, 136
Paris
  as an example to follow, 41, 51, 76
  Hygiene Conference (1889), 144
  life expectancy in 1878, 26
  as a threat to health, 7
  Sanitary Conference (1851), 20
  sewers and civilization in, 116
Parra, Félix, 98
Paso y Troncoso, Francisco del, 99
Paseo (*colonia*), 83
Paseo de la Reforma
  as center of power and memory, 79, 81
  costs of land and, 50
  as fashionable neighborhood, 52, 83, 84
  resources invested in, 86, 87 (table 5)
  as site of display of Porfirian state, xv
  as symbolic area, 91, 94–96, 100, 101, 104, 106, 141, 157
  urban landscape and, 77
Paseo de la Viga, 98, 101
Paseo del Emperador, 79, 80
Pasteur, Louis, 36, 37
Pearson and Sons, 86, 128
Pearson, Sir Weetman (Lord Cowdray), 127
Penal Code of 1872, 62
Penitentiary of San Lázaro, 49, 86, 87
Penitenciaría (*colonia*), 49
Peñafiel, Antonio, 28, 33–36, 89, 146
Peralvillo (*colonia*), 46, 51
pharmacies, 5, 59
pharmacists, 5
Plateros (street), 52
Plaza del Factor, 17
Plaza Mayor
  clearing of, 16
  as core of Tenochtitlán, 94
  first monument to Mexico's Independence (1864) and, 79
Plaza del Volador, 17
Popocatépetl (volcano), 88
Popular Hygiene Exhibition (Exposición Popular de Higiene, 1910), 113, 144–47. *See also* Centennial Celebrations of Mexico's Independence
Porfiriato, xii, xv, xviii, 19, 23, 47, 72, 76, 84–87, 88, 108, 155–56, 157–58
  criticisms towards, 113–14, 147, 150–52
  medical education during, 24
  national censuses during, 28
  positivism during, 25, 29, 39, 165n4
  Puebla during, 141–42
  Yucatán during, 142–43
  See also colonias, drainage, Mexico City, monuments, Porfirio Díaz, public health, statistics
Porter, Roy, 4
Prantl, Adolfo, 82
Protomedicato. *See* Royal Medical Board
public health
  definition of, 3

as a duty of the state, xv, 19, 20, 21, 22, 25, 29
education, 20, 21, 42, 56
idea of, 43, 75, 76, 78
ideas of modernity and progress and, 27, 30, 38–43
legislation, 15, 16, 19, 21
officials, 21, 22, 24–26, 28–31, 36, 43, 53, 56, 62, 68, 71, 72, 74, 75, 102, 111, 112, 115, 116, 124, 125, 132, 135, 137, 144, 149, 155
policies, xii, xv, 9; 4–6, 23, 31, 46, 47, 53, 54, 57–60, 102, 111, 112, 115, 116, 124, 125, 132, 135, 137, 148, 158
programs, 20, 24, 25, 29–31, 38–40, 47, 56–59, 62, 63, 69, 71, 72, 85, 87, 114, 117, 123, 125, 127, 128, 130–32, 134, 140, 143, 145, 146, 148, 150, 152, 153, 155, 158
sanitary movement and, 20, 29, 71
as a scientific discipline, 23
as a social and administrative science, 20, 29
and statistics, 24, 26–30, 38, 43, 74, 136, 144
See also sanitary code, Superior Sanitation Council
Puebla
influenza epidemic in, 142
measures to prevent cholera and typhus, 141, 142
sanitary conditions of, 141
urban improvements of, 142
Pulquerías, 68

Querétaro, 26
Quevedo, Miguel Angel de, 40, 41, 145
Quevedo y Zubieta, Salvador, 73, 74
Quintana Roo, 26

Rabasa, Emilio, 55
Raigosa, Genaro, 31–33, 37, 38
Ramírez, Joaquín, 98
Ramírez de Arellano, Nicolás, 133
Rastro (*colonia*), 46, 49, 52
Read and Campbell of London, 128
Rebull, Santiago, 79

Reform (historical period), 92, 94, 104, 105
Refugio (street), 52
Reglamento del Consejo Superior de Salubridad, 58
Resurrección (barrio), 127
Revillagigedo, Juan Vicente Güemez y Horcasitas – Segundo conde de, xv, xvi, 157
census of, 16
influence of, 18–19
nineteenth century reappraisal of, 1–2, 19
opposition to, 18
statue of, 1–2, 19
urban projects and, 2–3, 8, 15, 16, 17
Revolution of 1910. *See* Mexican Revolution
Reyes, Agustín , 26
Rincón Gallardo, Pedro, 125, 126, 139
Ringstrasse (Vienna, Austria), 80
Rio de Janeiro, 51
Riva Palacio, Vicente, 93, 95, 96, 97, 123
Rivas Góngora, Francisco, 126
Rivas Mercado, Antonio, 106
Rivera, Diego, 153
Robles, Carlos, 105
Rodríguez, Ida, 98
Rodríguez, José María, 153
Rodríguez Arangoity, Ramón, 79, 97
Roma (*colonia*), 46, 51, 83
Roma (street), 83
Rome, 14, 105, 116, 139
Romero, Matías, 130, 134
Romero Rubio (*colonia*), 46
Romero Rubio, Manuel, 128
Royal Medical Board (Protomedicato), 5, 20, 160n20
Ruiz, Luis E., 29, 39, 41, 145. *See also* hygienists

Saint John the Baptist (24th June), 69. *See also* bathing, urban poor, water
Saint Louis Missouri International Exhibition, 95
Salazar, Leopoldo, 103
San Álvaro (*colonia*), 46
San Cosme (*colonia*), 73
San Lázaro (barrio), 120, 138

San Lucas (market), 66
San Marco (piazza in Venice), 101
San Miguel Nonoalco (pueblo), 74
San Rafael (*colonia*), 46, 49
Sanitary Code of the State of New York, 61
Sanitary Code of the United States of Mexico (1891)
  lack of enforcement, 103
  reform of (1926), 153
  Sanitary administration of Mexico City, 61
  objectives of the 1891, 60–63
  origins of, 15, 16, 19, 21, 57
Sanitary Conference of 1851 (Paris), 20
sanitary engineering
  hygienists and, 24, 116
  mission of, 38, 43, 116
  public works and, 126, 155
sanitary inspectors, xiv-xv, xvi
  legal authority of, 62
  measures suggested by, 62–63, 70–73
  obstacles faced by, 71–72, 74, 75–76
  surveillance of the city and, 59–60, 63, 64, 72, 74, 75
  See also Sanitary Code of the United States of Mexico
sanitary science, 131
sanitary reform, 29, 142
Santa (novel character), 136–38
Santa Anna, 106. *See also* López de Santa Anna, Antonio
Santa Catarina (market), 66
Santa Julia (*colonia*), 46, 49
Santa María (*colonia*), 48–50, 73
Santiago Tlatelolco (customs building), 87
Santo Tomás (*colonia*), 46
Sarmiento, Domingo Faustino, 54, 74
Scheibe (*colonia*), 51
scientific journals, 21, 27, 60
scientific associations, 21, 39
Second Congress of Public Instruction 1890–91 (Mexico), 39
Secretaría de Comunicaciones y Obras Públicas (building), 84, 86, 87
Secretaría de Fomento, 120. *See also* Ministry of Economic Development

Sedano Francisco, 8, 16
sewers
  sewage system, 35, 130–33
  agriculture and, 133, 138
  combined sewer system, 131, 133–34
  complaints, 134–35
  disinfectants and, 123, 133
  inauguration of, 134
  literature and, 55, 137–38
  resources destined to, 86 (table 4), 134
  storm sewers, 130
  uncovered, 130
Sierra, Justo, 25, 27, 90, 96, 109
Sierra, Santiago, 27
Siliceo, Manuel, 120
Silva, Máximo, 147
Sociedad Mexicana de Geografía y Estadística, 28
Somera, Francisco, 80
Sonora, 142
Soriano, Manuel, 71–73
Sosa, Francisco, 96
Sosa, Secundino, 141
South America, 29
statistics, 26–30, 43, 74, 136, 144
  contradictory images of progress, 26, 27, 30, 74
  General Board of Statistics (Dirección General de Estadística), 27, 28
  infant mortality and, 26
  life expectancy, 26
  proofs of progress and, xii, 27, 29
  sanitary movement and, 28–30
  Superior Sanitation Council and, 27–28, 28–29
Stepan, Nancy Leys, 62
Stilwell Place (*colonia*), 83. *See also* Cuauhtémoc (*colonia*)
streets
  cleaning ordinances, 19, 53, 132
  conditions of, 11, 50, 54–55, 66, 68, 69, 134–35
  importance of paved, 6, 10, 39–40, 66, 86, 112, 131
  in Mérida, 142–43
  in Puebla, 141
  Plano ignográfico de la ciudad de México (1794), 17–18

Index

resources destined to pave the city's streets, 87 (table 5)
See also names of individual streets
Superior Sanitation Council (Consejo Superior de Salubridad)
 areas of concern, 57–62, 71, 103
 creation of, 21, 57–58
 Centennial Celebrations of Mexico's Independence and, 110–11, 144–45
 criticisms towards, 150
 drainage system and, 123, 124, 133
 Epidemiology Commission of, 62, 69
 germ theory of disease and, 37–38
 in 1917, 152–53
 Reglamento del Consejo Superior de Salubridad (1872), 56
 reorganization of (1879), 59–60
 Sanitary Code (1891) and, 60–62
 sanitary inspections of the city, 64–76
 sewage system and, 131, 133
 and use of statistics, 28, 30
 See also public health, sanitary inspectors

*T*acubaya (pueblo), 83
Tampico, 19, 86
Tehuantepec, 86
Teja (*colonia*), 46, 83
Teja (hacienda), 83
Tenango (river), 32
Tenenbaum, Barbara, 92
Tenochtitlán. See Mexico-Tenochtitlán
Tepic, 61
Tequixquiac (tunnel of), 140. See also drainage system
Thebes, 14
Tlalmanalco (river), 32
Tlalpan (pueblo), 111
Tlaxpana (*colonia*), 46
toilets, 101, 111
Tolsá, Manuel, 177n9
Tornel, José María, 53
Tula, 97
Tula (river), 117, 120, 121
Turner, John Kenneth, 143

*U*rban poor
 as carriers of disease, 68, 70, 71, 73, 75, 132, 149
 as immoral and backward, 30
 disorder among, 12
 lack of dress, 16, 113
 superstitious behavior, 23, 76, 132, 176n101
 vice-ridden, 13
 See also bathing, Mexico City
Uxmal, 97

*V*accination
 against rabies, 39, 64, 69
Valle Gómez (*colonia*), 46, 49, 112
Valley of Mexico
 drainage system and benefits to, 134, 139
 foundational past and, 31–33
 landscape of, 88
 Map of the Lakes in the Valley of Mexico, 121 (fig. 6)
Velasco, Francisco de, 142
Velasco, Ildefonso, 65
Velasco, José María, 88, 89
Velasco II, Luis de, viceroy, 117
Venice, 9, 101
Veracruz, 26, 81, 86, 95
Vienna, 80, 131
Viera, Juan de, 7
Vilar, Manuel, 98
Violante (*colonia*), 46, 48
Villarroel, Hipólito de, 2, 7, 11–13, 157
Volador (market), 66. See also Plaza del Volador

*W*arner, Marina, 99
Washington, D.C., 41
waste collection and disposal, 16, 53, 123, 130. See also sewers
water
 carriers, 41, 82
 circulation of, 17, 34
 distribution of, 28, 41, 102, 146, 192n118, 119

availability of drinking water, 28,
  41, 50, 51, 72, 74, 132, 146,
  192n118-119
expansion of the city and, 40, 48
polluted or tainted, 17, 32, 33, 34, 37,
  48, 53, 66, 69, 132–33
supply, 15, 102, 115, 143, 191n108
water-closets, 110, 111
See also aqueducts, bathing, disease
  causation, drainage, floods, sewers

Yellow fever
  in Buenos Aires, 54
  in Mexico City, 69
Yucatán, 142. *See also* Molina, Olegario

Zócalo, 79. *See also* Plaza Mayor
Zumpango (pueblo), 129, 140